Already published in BRACCO EDUCATION IN DIAGNOSTIC IMAGING

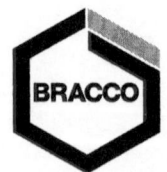

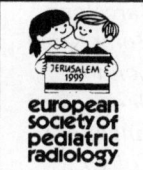

Springer

Milan
Berlin
Heidelberg
New York
Barcelona
Hong Kong
London
Paris
Singapore
Tokyo

Syllabus

HIGHLIGHTS OF PEDIATRIC RADIOLOGY

22nd Post-Graduate Course
European Society of Pediatric Radiology (ESPR)
Jerusalem, Israel, May 23-24, 1999

EDITORS:

J. BAR-ZIV

G. HOREV

G. KALIFA

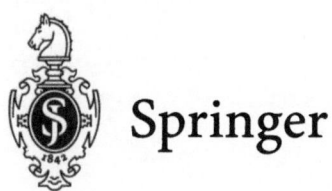 Springer

J. BAR-ZIV
Department of Radiology
Hadassah Medical Organization
Kiryat Hadassah
Jerusalem, Israel

G. HOREV
Department of Imaging
Schneider Children's Medical
Center of Israel
Petah-Tikva, Israel

G. KALIFA
Service de Radiologie
Hôpital Sain Vincent-de-Paul
Paris, France

© Springer-Verlag Italia, Milano 1999

ISBN 978-88-470-0061-2   ISBN 978-88-470-2253-9 (eBook)
DOI 10.1007/978-88-470-2253-9

Library of Congress Cataloging-in-Publication Data: applied for

Typesetting: Compostudio, Cernusco sul Naviglio (Milano)

SPIN: 10725709

Preface

Dear Colleagues,

 welcome to Jerusalem 1999 – an appropriate place for our professional gathering at the dawn of the coming millennium!

 An "All-Star" team of teachers is here for the Post-Graduate Course. They will focus on modern issues that are less frequently discussed at international conferences, emphasizing the radiological expression of patho-physiological processes. Lectures include topics on high resolution imaging in chest and abdomen, in bone and soft tissues. Discussions on pre- and post-therapy imaging will help underline our role in diagnosis and in therapy. This Syllabus includes detailed lecture manuscripts from the 22nd Post-Graduate Course.

 We would like to express our gratitude to the faculty of lecturers for their time and efforts, to the Bracco Company for sponsoring the Syllabus, and to Springer-Verlag for editing and printing this book.

May, 1999
J. Bar-Ziv
G. Horev
G. Kalifa (Editors)

Table of Contents

Session IV

SESSION I

SESSION 1

"Face Lifting" of the Newborn Chest-Surfactant and Extracorporeal Membrane Oxygenation

B. Newman

Department of Radiology, Children's Hospital of Pittsburgh, Pittsburgh, USA

Introduction

Important recent advances have been made in the management of newborn infants with respiratory distress. Few therapeutic maneuvers have had a greater impact than surfactant and extracorporeal membrane oxygenation (ECMO). Surfactant is a relatively inexpensive drug, administered quite easily through an endotracheal tube, and has had its greatest impact on the premature infant population in whom ECMO is usually contraindicated. Conversely, ECMO is a highly advanced, expensive, time and staff intensive, technically demanding procedure used mostly in full-term babies.

Surfactant

The successful clinical application of surfactant represents the most significant advance in neonatal care since the advent of positive pressure ventilation [1].

In the 1940s and '50s it was already recognized that neonates who died of "atelectasis" had very high alveolar surface tension and the suggestion was made to add surface active agents to correct this [1]. Surfactant was then isolated and characterized as a lipoprotein and shown to be deficient in hyaline membrane disease [1, 2]. Surprisingly its successful clinical use only occurred decades later. Early trials utilizing dipalmitoylphosphatidylcholine (DPPC), the major surface active lipid component of surfactant, showed no clinical benefit [3, 4]. It was later recognized that at least two hydrophobic surfactant apoproteins (SP-B and SP-C) were required to promote the adsorption and even thin spreading of the surfactant lipid component and resist inactivation of surfactant [1, 5, 6].

The first successful clinical use for surfactant was intratracheal administration of modified cow's lung surfactant in 1980 [7]. Currently surfactant agents in use include bovine and porcine agents derived from minced animal lungs or lung washings as well as several synthetic surfactants, which contain chemical protein substitutes. Work is underway in developing genetically engineered human surfactant [1].

Benefits of surfactant have included a prompt improvement in blood gas values and ventilatory settings with reduction in air leak phenomena as well as an overall decrease in neonatal mortality [8-12]. Benefits overall are similar with both synthetic and animal derived surfactants. The synthetic agents appear to be somewhat slower in initial action and more easily inactivated by intra-alveolar fluid but are cheaper and less likely to be contaminated [1, 13, 14].

The timing of the first surfactant dose is still controversial, i.e. prophylaxis or rescue. Early administration of surfactant has been shown to reduce morbidity and mortality in neonatal lung disease [13-15]. However, a large number of babies who would not have developed lung disease will incur the expense and risks of unnecessary treatment. Current conservative recommendations are that prophylactic administration of surfactant should be considered in all small babies less than 30 weeks who have the highest incidence of surfactant deficiency disease. Additionally, surfactant should be given as soon as possible once intubation is required [13, 15].

Multiple doses of surfactant are usually needed for a sustained clinical effect [1, 9, 13, 14, 16, 17]. Approximately three doses are given as an intratracheal bolus at 12 h intervals as required clinically. Surfactant is often administered as a bolus through an endotracheal tube with a side port so that ventilation can continue during installation. An alternative method that interrupts ventilation is administration via a catheter passed through the endotracheal tube. There are now special (and somewhat expensive) endotracheal tubes available with an intramural lumen that allows for deposition of surfactant beyond the endotracheal tip without interruption of ventilation. Surfactant administration is often associated with transient hypoxemia and hypercarbia thought to be related to temporary occlusion of the airway by the volume bolus [18, 19].

Despite careful administration, the distribution of surfactant is frequently uneven with resultant interspersed areas of residual atelectasis among reaerated portions of lung (Fig. 1) [20, 21]. Repeat dosing often takes care of this problem [17].

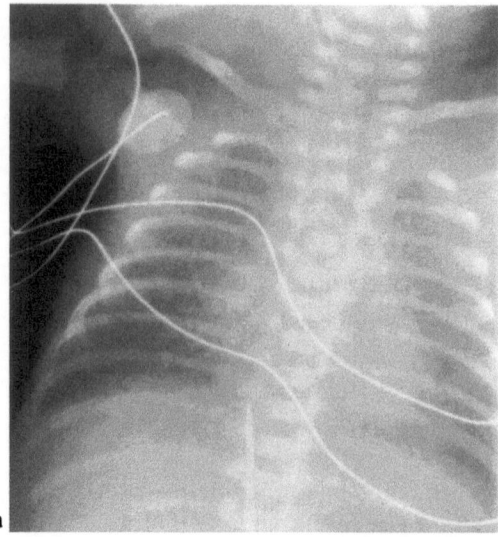

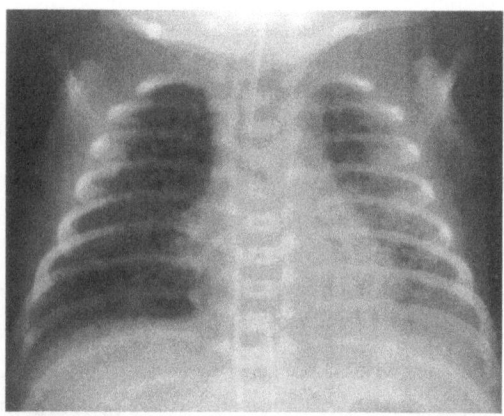

Fig. 1. a 28-week gestation newborn female infant with mild symmetric "ground glass" opacification of the lungs related to surfactant deficiency disease. **b** After 1 dose of surfactant there has been marked clearing of the lungs, greater on the right than the left. Pulmonary interstitial air has also developed possibly related to hyperventilation. In spite of high frequency ventilation this baby developed increased air leak and grade 4 intracranial hemorrhage and died

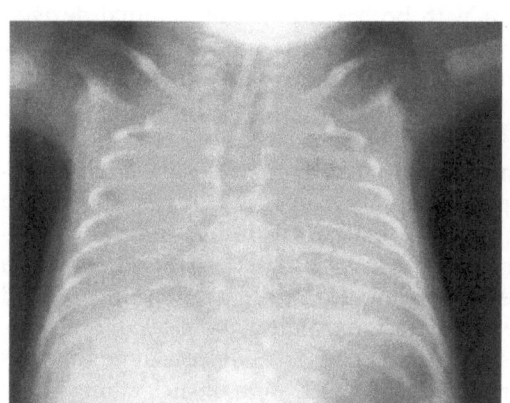

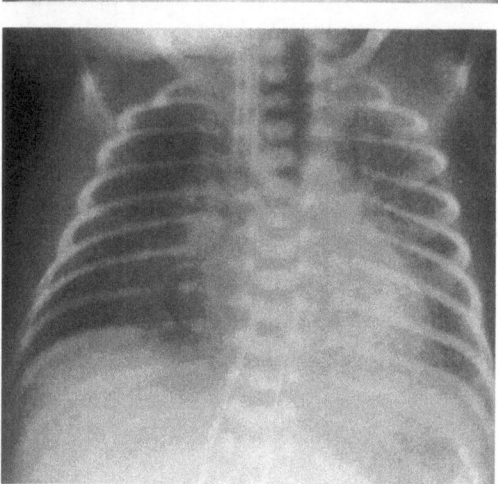

Fig. 2. a 26-week gestation male newborn infant-on an oscillating ventilator. There is marked diffuse pulmonary opacification due to surfactant deficiency ± fluid. Diffuse air bronchograms are present. **b** After two doses of surfactant there has been marked clearing with a more coarse pattern of opacification

The onset of action of surfactant is quite rapid [12]. As a result oxygen and ventilatory requirements need to be altered quickly to prevent hyperinflation, hyperoxia and interstitial air leak (Fig. 1) [9]. Surfactant is more effective in reducing surface tension when higher levels of positive end expiratory pressure (PEEP) and higher ventilatory rates are used [1]. Surfactant is more effective and longer lasting in larger babies perhaps because of the very marked degree of pulmonary immaturity in very tiny infants [12, 22, 23].

Radiographic changes after surfactant administration also occur quickly. Dramatic clearing of the lungs is often seen. The typical fine "ground glass" pattern is often transient, giving way to a coarse pattern as terminal airways distend (Fig. 2) [16, 20]. When sudden re-opacification of the lungs is seen radiographically differential considerations include: pulmonary edema, usually due either to abrupt increased left to right shunting through a patent ductus arteriosus (PDA) or neurogenic edema due to intraventricular hemorrhage; acute pulmonary hemorrhage seen mostly in very small premature infants and often also related to a PDA; or overaggressive ventilator reductions with recurrent atelectasis [20]. Development of interstitial emphysema after surfactant administration may be due to erroneous hyperventilation in relation to improving lung compliance and often results in a poor outcome (Fig. 1) [17].

Most small premature infants have a PDA. Typically, even before surfactant administration left to right shunting is present through the duct [18]. Rapid improvement in oxygenation such as occurs after surfactant administration leads to decreased pulmonary vascular resistance. Large left to right shunting can result in acute pulmonary edema and pulmonary hemorrhage [1, 24, 25]. The presence of pulmonary edema fluid necessitates higher ventilatory settings and also decreases the effectiveness of surfactant requiring larger and repeat drug dosage. Indomethacin is often used clinically to close the ductus and prevent this problem.

The incidence of bronchopulmonary dysplasia (BPD) was expected to be reduced by the use of surfactant, but has disappointingly not significantly changed [11, 12]. This has been attributed to an increase in survival of very tiny premature infants with a very high risk of

BPD. The overall severity of BPD has been appreciably decreased, especially in larger babies [1].

In general surfactant has been a safe agent with few problems. The modified animal surfactant proteins are only about 80% homologous with the human sequence. As a result antibodies to the foreign proteins are a potential risk, especially in older immunocompetent babies [1]. Antibody formation to surfactant has been documented with exogenous surfactant administration and post-lung transplantation in babies with congenital surfactant protein B deficiency, although no harmful clinical effects were apparent [26]. In addition, a small increase in sepsis has also been identified especially with the animal-based surfactant agents [1]. Increased pulmonary hemorrhage and mucus plugging have been attributed to both types of surfactant [1].

Before the availability of surfactant, prenatal steroid use had been shown to be beneficial in reducing neonatal mortality, pulmonary disease, interventricular hemorrhage and necrotizing enterocolitis [27, 28]. After the widespread use of surfactant, research studies have shown that steroids and surfactant have a synergistic benefit so that the availability of surfactant should not obviate the appropriate use of prenatal steroids [1, 28].

Surfactant has been further shown to be useful in conditions other than primary surfactant deficiency in premature infants. Babies with meconium aspiration syndrome show improvement with administration of surfactant. It is thought that the meconium may inactivate surfactant as well as cause secondary surfactant deficiency due to hypoxic injury to surfactant producing cells [14, 29].

Congenital diaphragmatic hernia patients are also deficient in surfactant. Administration of surfactant has been shown to improve oxygenation and decrease the need for ECMO and time on ECMO in these and other full term babies [14, 19, 30, 31].

Interestingly, surfactant is not effective treatment for congenital protein B deficiency. The reasons for this are unclear, possibilities include abnormal protein phospholipid proportions, defective cellular uptake and resecretion of surfactant, abnormal protein C and other surfactant components and possible antibody formation [26].

Extracorporeal Membrane Oxygenation

In spite of numerous effective therapeutic options, such as surfactant, nitric oxide, pre and postnatal steroids and new ventilatory techniques such as high frequency respirators, there are still many neonates who will die of respiratory failure unless an alternative method of oxygenation is available [32]. In addition, aggressive ventilator therapy carries a high price in terms of morbidity and chronic lung disease. Hence the search to develop a safe, prolonged external circuit bypass technique for the cardiorespiratory support of selected newborn infants.

Early cardiopulmonary bypass equipment utilized a bubble oxygenator, which directly exposed blood to oxygen and rapidly damaged blood cells and proteins, especially with prolonged bypass [32]. The solution to this problem and a major step towards ECMO was the development of a membrane oxygenator in which there is no direct blood gas interface. Silicone became the standard membrane material because of its excellent gas transfer properties. Once the membrane and circuits were coated with a protein monolayer, blood was no longer in contact with a thrombogenic foreign surface, allowing gas exchange to occur for a prolonged period of time without causing excess damage to blood cells [32].

Various types of pumps were developed for ECMO use, these have attempted to minimize hemolysis, and prevent air access while being able to be used over a wide range of flows. All of the current pumps, however, provide nonpulsatile systemic flow [32].

Vascular access was an additional problem to overcome. Initially attempts were made to use umbilical vessels; however, these did not provide adequate flow for total cardiorespiratory support. Ultimately the internal jugular vein and common carotid artery proved to be the best sites. The initial successful neonatal application of ECMO occurred in 1975 [33]. Since that time ECMO use has become widespread in major medical centers.

ECMO is typically used when severe respiratory disease is thought to be reversible. Indications include meconium aspiration syndrome, pneumonia, sepsis, primary pulmonary hypertension, congenital diaphragmatic hernia, asphyxia, respiratory distress syndrome, barotrauma with air leak and perioperative support of newborns with congenital heart disease (Figs. 3, 4) [25, 30, 34, 35]. Occasionally ECMO is utilized for other conditions that may mimic pulmonary hypertension such as obstructed total anomalous pulmonary venous return, pulmonary hypoplasia and congenital surfactant B deficiency.

Selection of patients for ECMO has been the subject of considerable controversy. Ideal selection criteria would predict which infants would do poorly on mechanical ventilation before they have life-threatening complications or irreversible lung disease. Many centers use a numeric scoring system to estimate mortality rate and utilize ECMO when the predicted mortality is greater than 80% [25, 32, 36]. However, patients should not be so moribund that they will no longer benefit from ECMO. Sudden acute irreversible deterioration in cardiorespiratory status and significant barotrauma have become additional indicators for ECMO use [32, 37].

ECMO contraindications include situations in which the patient is unlikely to have a high quality outcome or ECMO cannot be achieved without unacceptable morbidity [25, 32, 38]. This includes small premature infants, less than 2 000 g, who have a very high risk of intraventricular hemorrhage, this risk is much increased on EC-

MO due to the requirement for complete anticoagulation. ECMO can still be utilized in infants who have had small grade 1 or grade 2 intraventricular hemorrhages, hemorrhage greater than this is considered a contraindication to ECMO. Infants with severe chromosomal aberrations or syndromes associated with profound mental retardation or typical fatal outcome should also be excluded from ECMO therapy. Research is currently being done on ECMO in smaller infants using heparin bonded circuits that avoid systemic anticoagulation.

Prior to institution of ECMO, echocardiography is performed to evaluate for intrinsic cardiac defects and pulmonary hypertension. Ultrasound is usually done to evaluate the head and presence of intracranial hemorrhage. An electroencephalograph is performed to assess hypoxic ischemic encephalopathy. Attention must be paid to optimal placement of tubes and catheters prior to ECMO as later manipulation is undesirable due to systemic anticoagulation.

Two forms of ECMO bypass are available. The most commonly utilized is double cannula venoarterial bypass. A new and less common technique is either double cannula or single cannula, double lumen venovenous bypass techniques (Table 1) (Fig. 3).

In venoarterial bypass (Fig. 4) venous blood is removed from the right atrium via a catheter in the inter-

Table 1. Comparison of venoarterial and venovenous ECMO (Modified from [32])

Venoarterial ECMO	Venovenous ECMO
Complete cardiorespiratory support	No cardiac support
Carotid artery ligation	Sparing of carotid artery
Decreased pulmonary blood flow	Normal pulmonary flow and perfusion
Lower O_2 delivery to myocardium	Normal perfusion of myocardium
Higher PO_2 (potential for hyperoxia)	Lower PO_2 levels
Can use smaller catheters	Single double lumen catheter, limited to larger babies
Higher incidence of vascular thrombosis	No arterial thrombotic complications
Extensive clinical experience	Limited clinical experience

nal jugular vein. Externally oxygenated blood is returned to the aortic arch through a cannula in the right common carotid artery. This method allows complete cardiorespiratory support.

Venovenous ECMO provides respiratory support

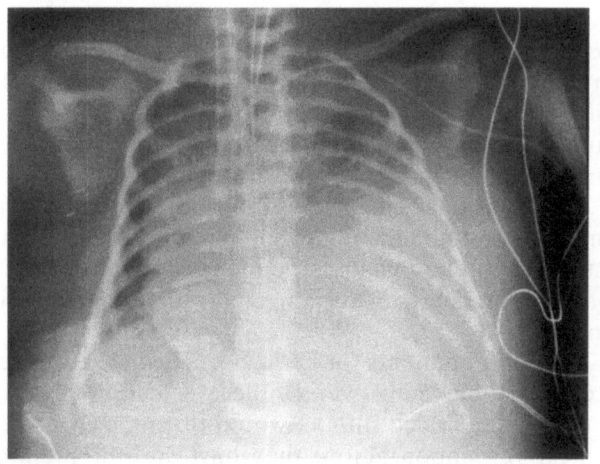

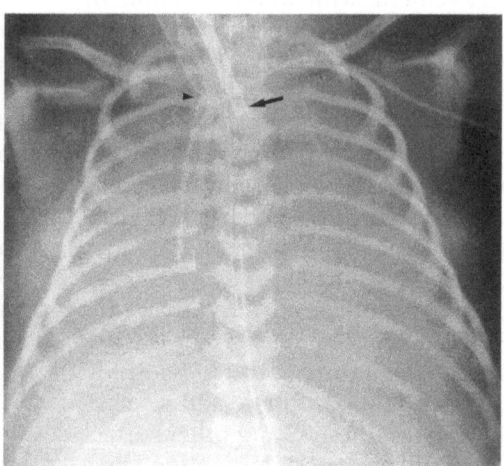

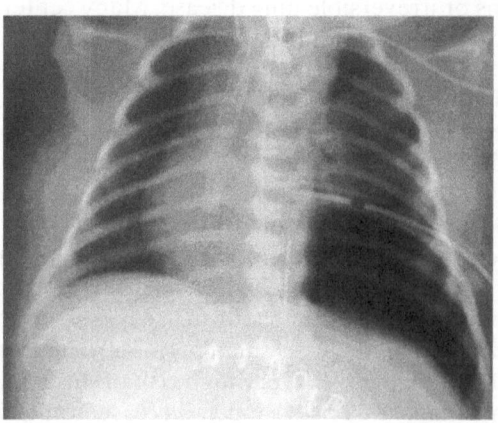

Fig. 3 a-c. *Male infant with unrepaired left congenital diaphragmatic hernia.* **a** Venovenous ECMO was initiated on day 4 of life. The large single cannula with multiple side ports has been inserted in the right jugular vein with the tip slightly high in the right atrium. An additional left subclavian/right atrial central line is in place as well as the endotracheal tube, nasogastric tube and umbilical arterial line. There is opacity in the left upper and lower chest (atelectasis and hernia) and rightward cardiomediastinal shift with patchy right atelectasis. There is moderate anasarca. **b** 3 days later the baby required conversion to venoarterial ECMO due to cardiac decompensation with placement of the arterial cannula through the right carotid artery to the aortic arch (*arrow*). The lungs are deaerated and diffusely opaque. Note that the venous catheter is moderately kinked (*arrowhead*). **c** Repair of diaphragmatic hernia on ECMO day 9. There is a collapsed hypoplastic left lung and large left pneumothorax. The right lung is clear. The baby was weaned off ECMO 1 day later

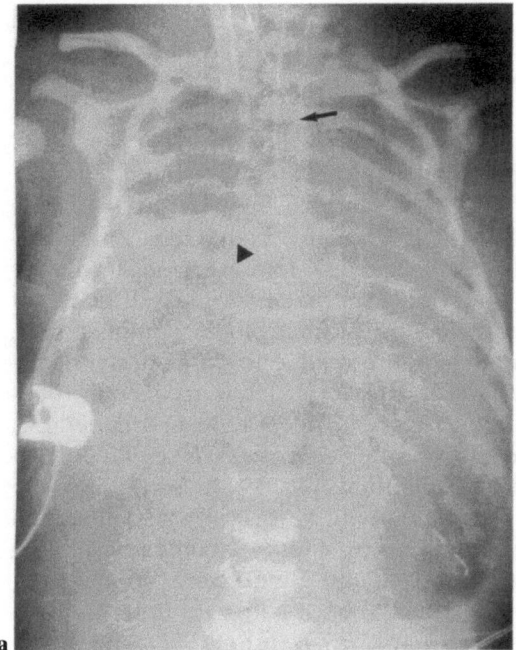

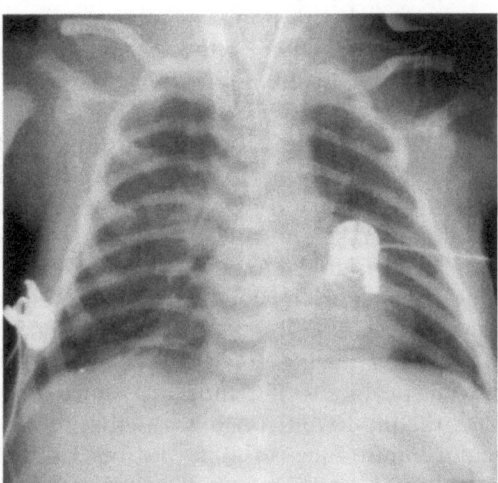

Fig. 4 a, b. *Full-term male infant placed on venoarterial ECMO for meconium aspiration.* **a** The arterial cannula tip is at the level of the aortic arch (*arrow*). The distal portion of the venous catheter is not radio-opaque and therefore not visible. The tip of the venous catheter in the right atrium is visible as a small radiopaque dot (*arrowhead*). Note the diffusely opacified deaerated lungs. **b** 5 days later-improved pulmonary aeration with patchy pulmonary opacities presumably residua of aspiration pneumonia. The baby was in the process of being weaned off ECMO

and blood oxygenation but relies on the infant heart to support the systemic circulation. Venous outflow is still via the internal jugular vein and venous return usually via the femoral vein. With the newer double lumen catheter the internal jugular vein is used alone with separate outflow and return ports (Fig. 3). Patient size is a limiting factor in the single catheter technique as the catheter used is 14 F or larger [39]. Mild or moderate cardiac decompensation will often reverse with venovenous ECMO support because of enhanced myocardial oxygenation, decreased lung hyperinflation and improved systemic circulation [39]. The efficacy and safety of the two ECMO techniques appear to be similar [32, 39, 40]. The advantage of the venous technique is that the carotid artery is not utilized, sparing the neonate any possible consequences of manipulation or ligation of this vessel (Table 1) [41]. However, patients on venovenous ECMO may be a greater management challenge and may require conversion to venoarterial ECMO if cardiac failure develops (Fig. 3).

Early in the course of ECMO little or no oxygenation occurs in the infant's lungs and circuit flow is around 100-120 ml/kg per min [32]. Ventilator settings are typically kept very low to allow the lungs to rest, in order to facilitate recovery. The lungs tend to be underaerated and opacified reflecting a combination of underlying lung disease, atelectasis and capillary leak edema (Figs. 3b and 4a) [42, 43]. There is a current tendency to maintain higher levels of PEEP during ECMO so that the lungs become less deaerated. This allows better lung compliance and appears to shorten the course of ECMO.

While on ECMO, frequent chest radiographs, often daily, are obtained to assess catheter position and evalu-

ate the lungs. Serial head ultrasounds and echocardiograms are done to evaluate intracranial hemorrhage and intracerebral blood flow and assess cardiac function, pulmonary hypertension and ductal shunting. Complete nutritional support is established, usually with hyperalimentation. Prophylactic antibiotics are given in conjunction with ECMO. Respiratory therapy and pulmonary suction are performed frequently and normocapnia is maintained to stimulate respiratory effort and maintain respiratory muscle tone.

As the infant's pulmonary status improves, increasing oxygenation takes place via the lungs allowing flow through the external circuit to be reduced according to need (Fig. 4b). Weaning is accomplished by slowly decreasing the flow to about 50-80 ml per min. If the baby remains stable the catheters are clamped and then removed several hours later. With decannulation from venoarterial ECMO, the carotid artery used for arterial access is most often ligated. In some centers repair and reanastomosis of the artery is attempted [41]. There are concerns about stenosis, dissection or pseudoaneurysm at the repair site and the potential for future thromboembolic disease [29].

While on ECMO there is a general increase in extracellular fluid manifested often by increased extra-axial fluid on head ultrasound and body wall edema on radiographs (Fig. 3a). Lasix diuresis is frequently utilized and may also help shorten ECMO time [44].

ECMO complications include those related to mechanical failure and patient complications. [30, 32, 36, 42, 45] ECMO is a highly demanding technique requiring considerable specialty training and expertise. Technical problems in this environment are fortunately rare though when they occur it may be disastrous [32]. The rate of oxygenator failure is quite small, approximately 4%. Rupture of tubing or a tear in the tubing or membrane with resultant hemorrhage or air embolism is the most serious technical concern while clot formation in the circuit is the most common problem [45]. Cannula malposition problems may be associated with poor venous outflow, disruption, damage or dissection of the jugular vein or carotid artery and massive bleeding [45]. Arterial cannula malposition too close to the aortic valve may cause valvular insufficiency, dysfunction or disruption. Distal placement of the arterial cannula can lead to compromised cerebral and coronary flow [32, 45]. Vessel thrombosis or pseudoaneurysms during or after ECMO are additional vascular complications related to ECMO. They appear to occur more frequently with venoarterial than venovenous ECMO [39].

Patient complications are common during ECMO and include both acute and chronic problems. The most common of these is hemorrhage related to anticoagulation [25, 32, 38, 45]. Of particular importance is the occurrence of intracranial hemorrhage. A combination of factors may predispose to intracranial hemorrhage, the most important are thought to be anticoagulation, preexisting ischemia, venous hypertension related to jugular vein ligation [46] and potential for air or thrombotic emboli [46]. Hemorrhage does not always occur in predictable sites, there appears to be a predisposition for posterior fossa bleeding. On sonography hemorrhage may be hypoechoic or of mixed echogenicity perhaps because of anticoagulation [38]. Bleeding at the neck incision sites and other previous surgical sites can also be significant. Pleural and pericardial hemorrhage may be difficult to recognize when the lungs are generally opaque. The presence of mediastinal shift may be helpful and ultrasound may be of use when the lungs are opacified. Bleeding complications can be treated by a decrease in heparin infusion and transfusion of platelets. Sometimes discontinuation of ECMO is required. Occasionally surgical intervention may be required. Surgical procedures such as repair of congenital diaphragmatic hernia can be performed while on ECMO with appropriate boosting of platelets and blood product replacement (Fig. 3c).

Systolic hypertension is a serious side effect of ECMO. Renal failure occurs in about 10% of patients on ECMO and can be treated with addition of a hemofilter to the ECMO circuit. There is a risk of infection that increases with longer duration of cardiac bypass. Prophylactic antibiotics and constant surveillance are required. Other ECMO complications include cholestasis, likely related to hyperalimentation and splenomegaly thought to be due to sequestration of damaged red blood cells and platelets. Patients with prolonged chest wall edema have a tendency to develop diffuse periosteal reaction around the ribs [38].

Pulmonary edema probably due to capillary leak is common for a variable time post-ECMO. Bronchopulmonary dysplasia does occur in patients who have been on ECMO and is correlated with delayed institution or very prolonged ECMO [47]. It appears that ECMO has a somewhat protective effect on the lungs or at least is not associated with an increased risk of BPD.

Intracranial abnormalities on ultrasound and CT imaging are common both during and after ECMO treatment [48, 49]. Low birth weight, sepsis and prolonged ECMO are risk factors. However, long term neurologic follow up indicates that ECMO itself does not increase the incidence of neurologic complications, These appear to be more related to the underlying disease that necessitates ECMO [29]. Initial concerns related to carotid artery ligation appear to be unfounded [32, 50]. Neurodevelopmental outcomes are similar in ECMO and non-ECMO infants [38, 48].

ECMO is associated with an overall survival rate of approximately 81%, an excellent outcome considering that this is a group of patients almost certain to die without ECMO. Outcome has been better for meconium aspiration and pulmonary hypertension (93%) than congenital diaphragmatic hernia (58%) [29, 32].

The objectives of ECMO, to circumvent the lungs, protect the lungs from high pressure ventilation and oxygen toxicity and allow them to heal appear to have been attained. Additionally, simply having ECMO as a final resort has enabled greater experimentation with other techniques and development of alternative methods of managing severe respiratory distress with resultant recent decreased use of ECMO [29]. Therapeutic alternatives include inhaled nitric oxide, high frequency ventilation and the use of permissive hypercapnia in diaphragmatic hernia patients. Care must be taken however, to use other therapeutic options judiciously and make the decision to move to ECMO at an appropriate time before irreversible brain and lung injury occur [29].

References

1. Long WA, Guangbin Z, Henry GW (1996) Pharmacologic adjuncts II: exogenous surfactants. In: Goldsmith JP, Karotkin EH (eds) Assisted ventilation of the neonate, 3rd edn. WB Saunders, Philadelphia, pp 305-325
2. Avery ME, Mead J (1959) Surface active properties in relation to atelectasis and hyaline membrane disease. Am J Dis Child 17: 517-523
3. Chu J, Clements JA, Cotton EK, et al. (1967) Neonatal pulmonary ischemia. Part 1: clinical and physiological studies. Pediatrics 40: 709-782
4. Robillard E, Alaire Y, Dagenais-Perusse P, et al. (1964) Microaerosol administration of synthectic beta-gamma-dipalmitoyl-L-alpha-lecithin in the respiratory distress syndrome: a preliminary report. Can Med Assoc J 90: 55-57
5. Hawgood S, Clements JA (1990) Surfactant and its apoproteins. J Clin Invest 86: 1
6. Soll RF (1997) Surfactant therapy in the USA: trials and current routines. Biol Neonate 71(Suppl 1): 1-7
7. Fujiwara T, Chida S, Watabe Y, et al. (1980) Artificial surfactant therapy in hyaline membrane disease. Lancet 1: 55-59
8. Hennes HM, Lee MB, Rimm AA, Shapiro DL (1991) Sur-

factant replacement therapy in respiratory distress syndrome. AJDC 145: 102-104

9. Dunn MS, Shennan AT, Possmayer F (1990) Single-versus multiple-dose surfactant replacement therapy in neonates of 30-36 weeks' gestation with respiratory distress syndrome. Pediatrics 86: 564-571

10. Phibbs RH, Ballard RA, Clements JA, Heilbron DC, Phibbs CS, Schlueter MA, et al. (1991) Initial clinical trial of EXO-SURF, a protein-free synthetic surfactant, for the prophylaxis and early treatment of Hyaline membrane disease. Pediatrics 88: 1-9

11. Jobe AH (1993) Pulmonary surfactant therapy. N Engl J Med 328: 861-868

12. McColley SA (1998) Bronchopulmonary dysplasia. Impact of surfactant replacement therapy. Pediatr Clin North Am 45: 573-585

13. Kattwinkel J (1998) Surfactant: evolving issues. Clin Perinatol 25: 17-32

14. Soll RF (1996) Appropriate surfactant usage in 1996. Eur J Pediatr 155(Suppl 2): 8-13

15. Morley CJ (1997) Systematic review of prophylactic vs rescue surfactant. Arch Dis Child 77: F70-F74

16. Schimmel MS (1995) Respiratory distress syndrome: therapeutic aspects. Pediatr Radiol 25: 641-642

17. Dinger J, Schwarze R, Rupprecht E (1997) Radiological changes after therapeutic use of surfactant in infants with respiratory distress syndrome. Pediatr Radiol 27: 26-31

18. Skinner JR (1997) The effects of surfactant on haemodynamics in hyaline membrane disease. Arch Dis Child Fetal Neonatal Ed 76: F67-F69

19. Lotze A, Mitchell BR, Bulas DI, Zola EM, Shalwitz RA, Gunkel JH, et al. (1998) Multicenter study of surfactant (beractant) use in the treatment of term infants with severe respiratory failure. J Pediatr 132: 40-47

20. Cleveland RH (1995) A radiologic update on medical diseases of the newborn chest. Pediatr Radiol 25: 631-637

21. Dimitriou G, Greenough A, Griffin FJ, Karani J (1995) The appearance of "early" chest radiographs and the response to surfactant replacement therapy. Br J Radiol 68: 1177-1180

22. Swischuk LE, Shetty BP, John SD (1996) The lungs in immature infants: how important is surfactant therapy in preventing chronic lung problems? Pediatr Radiol 26: 508-511

23 Soll RF (1998) Surfactant treatment of the very preterm infant. Biol Neonate 74(Suppl 1): 35-42

24. Clyman RI, Jobe A, Heymann M, Ikegami M, Roman C, Payne B, et al. (1982) Increased shunt through the patent ductus arteriosus after surfactant replacement therapy. J Pediatr 100: 101-107

25. Wood BP (1993) The newborn chest. Radiol Clin North Am 31: 667-676

26. Hamvas A, Nogee LM, Mallory GB Jr., Spray TL, Huddleston CB, August A, et al. (1997) Lung transplantation for treatment of infants with surfactant protein B deficiency. J Pediatr 130: 231-239

27. Goetzman BW, Milstein JM (1996) Pharmacologic adjuncts I. In: Goldsmith JP, Karotkin EH (eds) Assisted ventilation of the neonate. WB Saunders, Philadelphia, pp 296-300

28. Northway WH (1992) Bronchopulmonary dysplasia: twenty-five years later. Pediatrics 89: 969-973

29. Kanto WP Jr, Bunyapen C (1998) Extracorporeal membrane oxygenation. Controversies in selection of patients and management. Clin Perinatol 25: 123-135

30. Langer JC (1998) Congenital diaphragmatic hernia. Chest Surg Clin N Am 8: 295-314

31. Stillerman LR, Gunn SB, Hart JC, Engle WA (1997) Effects of exogenous surfactant on neonates supported by extracorporeal membrane oxygenation. J Perinatol 17: 262-265

32. Torosian MB, Statter MB, Arensman RM (1996) Extracorporeal membrane oxygenation. In: Goldsmith JP, Karotkin EH, (eds) Assisted ventilation of the neonate, 3rd edn. WB Saunders, Philadelphia, pp 241-256

33. Bartlett RH, Gazzaniga AB, Jefferies MR, et al. (1976) Extracorporeal membrane oxygenation (ECMO) cardiopulmonary support in infancy. Trans Am Soc Artif Intern Organs 22: 80-93

34. Fox WW, Dura S (1983) Persistent pulmonary hypertension in the neonate: diagnosis and management. J Pediatr 103: 505-514

35. Bartlett RH, Toomasian J, Roloff D, et al. (1986) Extracorporeal membrane oxygenation in neonatal respiratory failure: 100 cases. Ann Surg 204: 236-245

36. Short BL, Miller MK, Anderson KD (1987) Extracorporeal membrane oxygenation in the management of respiratory failure in the newborn. Clin Perinatol 14: 737-748

37. Redmond CR, Graves ED, Falterman KW, et al. (1987) Extracorporeal membrane oxygenation for respiratory and cardiac failure in infants and children. J Thorac Cardiovasc Surg 93: 199-204

38. Swischuk LE (1997) Imaging of the newborn, infant, and young child, 4th edn. Williams & Wilkins, Baltimore, pp 105-107

39. Knight GR, Dudell GG, Evans ML, Grimm PS (1996) A comparison of venovenous and venoarterial extracorporeal membrane oxygenation in the treatment of neonatal respiratory failure. Crit Care Med 24: 1678-1683

40. Cornish JD, Heiss KF, Clark RH, et al. (1993) Efficacy of venovenous extracorporeal membrane oxygenation for neonates with respiratory and circulatory compromise. J Pediatr 122: 105-109

41. DeAngelis GA, Mitchell DG, Merton DA, Wolfson PJ, Desai HJ, Desai SA, et al. (1992) Right common carotid artery reconstruction in neonates after extracorporeal membrane oxygenation: color Doppler imaging. Radiology 182: 521-525

42. Gross GW, Cullen J, Kornhauser MS, Wolfson PJ (1992) Thoracic complications of extracorporeal membrane oxygenation: findings on chest radiographs and sonograms. AJR 158: 353-358

43. Taylor GA, Short BL, Kriesmer P (1986) Extracorporeal membrane oxygenation: radiographic appearance of the neonatal chest. AJR 146: 1257-1260

44. Kelly RE, Phillips JD, Foglia RP, et al. (1991) Pulmonary edema and fluid mobilization as determinants of the duration of ECMO support. J Pediatr Surg 26: 1016-1022

45. Zwischenberger JB, Nguyen TT, Upp JR Jr, et al. (1994) Complications of neonatal extracorporeal membrane oxygenation. Collective experience from the Extracorporeal Life Support Organization. J Thorac Cardiovasc Surg 107: 838-848

46. Weber TR, Kountzman B (1996) The effects of venous occlusion on cerebral blood flow characteristics during ECMO. J Pediatr Surg 31: 1124-1127

47. Kornhauser MS, Cullen JA, Baumgart S, et al. (1994) Risk factors for bronchopulmonary dysplasia after extracorporeal membrane oxygenation. Arch Pediatr Adolesc Med 148: 820-825

48. Graziani LJ, Gringlas M, Baumgart S (1997) Cerebrovascular complications and neurodevelopmental sequelae of neonatal ECMO. Clin Perinatol 24: 655-675

49. Bulas DI, Taylor GA, O'Donnell RM, Short BL, Fitz CR, Vezina G (1996) Intracranial abnormalities in infants treated with extracorporeal membrane oxygenation: update on sonographic and CT findings. AJNR 17: 287-294

50. Hofkosh D, Thompson AE, Nozza RJ, et al. (1991) Ten years of extracorporeal membrane oxygenation: neurodevelopmental outcome. Pediatrics 87: 549-555

Airways Obstruction in Children

H. Carty

Department of Radiology, Alder Hey Children's Hospital, Liverpool, England

Introduction

Airways obstruction in children may present acutely, dramatically and fatally, but more commonly has a gradual onset with chronic or progressive symptoms. General principles underpinning the major considerations will be reviewed. The lesions that cause airways obstruction in children are briefly outlined.

Symptoms

Acute. Acute airways obstruction is rare. The infant or child presents with rapid onset of noisy distressed breathing, stridor and as hypoxia occurs, cyanosis and death if relief is not obtained. The most frequent cause of this is inhalation of a foreign body with total tracheal obstruction, or laryngeal oedema caused by trauma or allergy.

Intermediate. Symptoms are similar. The child presents with a history of stridor, tachypnoea, noisy distressed breathing. The length of history depends on the cause and will range from hours to days. There may be a history of difficulty in breathing during eating such as occurs with choanal atresia, or drooling at the mouth with difficulty in swallowing as is the case with retropharyngeal abscesses, or epiglottitis. The radiological investigation of such children depends on the suspected cause and will range from none to the use of magnetic resonance imaging (MRI).

Chronic. Children with chronic airways obstruction present most frequently with the effects of hypoxaemia: narcolepsy, Pickwickian syndrome and Ondine's curse, and ultimately pulmonary hypertension. Milder forms of this are manifest by snoring, attention deficit and poor performance at school. Less dramatically, disorder may present with speech or feeding difficulties due to obstruction by enlarged tonsils. The failure to eat normally may lead to failure to thrive and growth arrest.

Imaging

Magnetic Resonance

All children with suspected tumour or neurogenic causes of airways obstruction should be imaged by MRI with images taken in the coronal and axial plane. T1 and T2 weighted sequences and a fat suppression technique are required. Gadolinium enhancement is required for tumors. MR is the preferred cross sectional imaging technique for full mapping of neck masses such as lymphangiomas even if these are also assessed with ultrasound. MR imaging of mediastinal masses and suspected vascular anomalies is well-established. For tumors such as rhabdomyosarcoma that have bone destruction in addition to the soft tissue component, the MR should be supplemented by computed tomography (CT).

Computed Tomography

With the advent of MR, the role of CT in imaging tumors as a cause of airways obstruction has diminished. Its main indication today is in the imaging of bone destruction and the rare tumors that cause obstruction. It remains the method of choice for imaging choanal atresia to localise the extent of the bony bar prior to surgery. CT of the lungs is required for the demonstration of pulmonary metastases. Radiographs supplemented as deemed appropriate by CT in both coronal and axial planes are required to identify the extent of the bony deformity in congenital facial malformations that lead to airways obstruction such as hemifacial microsomia. CT is also the technique of choice in trauma. Spiral CT of the trachea with 3D reconstruction has been shown to demonstrate tracheomalacia without the need for bronchoscopy.

Cross-sectional imaging must be done properly. Movement artefact can cause diagnostic errors both by overdiagnosing or missing lesions; therefore many children will need sedation. In children with a compromised airway, oral sedation may not be safe and it is preferable that these children are imaged during intubated anaesthesia.

Ultrasound

Ultrasound is a helpful initial screening investigation of the neck or anterior mediastinal masses. These can be rapidly characterised as solid or cystic and the relationship to major vessels identified. An assessment can be made as to whether ultrasound-guided biopsy is feasible. Ultrasound imaging of the vocal cords and subglottic region can be done dynamically, the infant being kept quiet by sucking on a soother dipped in glycerine. Ultrasound provides a non-invasive method of screening for vocal cord lesions such as haemangiomas or lymphangiomas and vocal cord movement. High frequency linear array probes are required. These need to be small enough to deal with the small size of the child's neck.

Radiographs

The role of conventional radiography in trying to identify the extent of lesions in the face, head and neck is now obsolete. A lateral radiograph of the post nasal space (PNS) is however the simplest, cheapest and quickest method of assessing the adenoids as a possible cause of airways obstruction and is indicated when appropriate. This must be a good quality straight film in the true lateral position. Digital radiographs are preferable to standard films.

The lateral radiograph should also be the first imaging investigation in suspected retropharyngeal abscess, or opaque foreign body inhalation. Children with clear clinical evidence of acute infective causes of airways obstruction such as croup or epiglottitis do not require airways imaging and it may be dangerous, especially in children with epiglottitis who can obstruct very suddenly. A chest X-ray may be required in children with croup who have persistent lower tract signs and do not recover as clinically expected. The lateral X-ray must be truly lateral, as obliquity causes superimposition of structure, which may lead to a mistaken diagnosis of pathology. Due to the laxity of laryngeal structure, the subglottic regions may "collapse" during inspiration causing apparent subglottic stenosis. Films taken in head flexion and expiration can cause marked thickening of the retropharyngeal tissues simulating a retropharyngeal abscess. This is even more pronounced if the child is crying. On a repeat view with the neck extended this thickening will disappear.

Sinus radiographs in addition to the PNS view are frequently requested in children presenting with airways obstruction to identify sinus disease. The maxillary antra do not become adequately pneumatized until about 4 years of age to render them visible radiographically. Mucosal thickening and sinus opacity cannot be assessed adequately before this. In older children a simple 30° occipitomental (O.M.) view done PA to protect the eyes from the primary beam is all that is required. The finding of mucosal thickening should be related to symptoms. There is a great variability in the incidence of mucosal thickening in the population. Such thickening is a frequent incidental finding on routine MR. The preferred method for looking for ostial obstruction as a cause of recurrent sinus disease thought to be exacerbating upper airways obstruction is coronal CT.

Fluoroscopy

Contrast studies are the initial investigation in suspected vascular anomalies and in children who have had surgery for repair of tracheo oesophageal fistula who develop upper airways obstruction due to compression of the trachea by a distended proximal pouch, or have severe tracheomalacia. While this latter is better imaged by bronchoscopy, a collapsing trachea may also be seen during fluoroscopy. Ideally, the fluoroscopic studies should be recorded on video to allow review.

The obstructing lesions

Full descriptions of the lesions outlined in the Tables can be found in standard textbooks. A brief outline of the salient features is given here. The causes of upper airways tract obstruction are shown in Table 1.

Choanal atresia

This condition has a probable frequency of in 18 000 live births. Females are twice as likely to be affected as males. Bilateral atresia is rare; it is mostly unilateral and is usually discovered by failure to pass a naso-gastric tube through the nostril. Bilateral disease presents with mouth breathing and difficulty in feeding as the child cannot breathe while a bottle teat is in the mouth. This presents in the neonatal period. Unilateral atresia can present at any age.

Contrast instilled into a nostril normally passes freely into the nasopharynx. In choanal atresia, due to the ob-

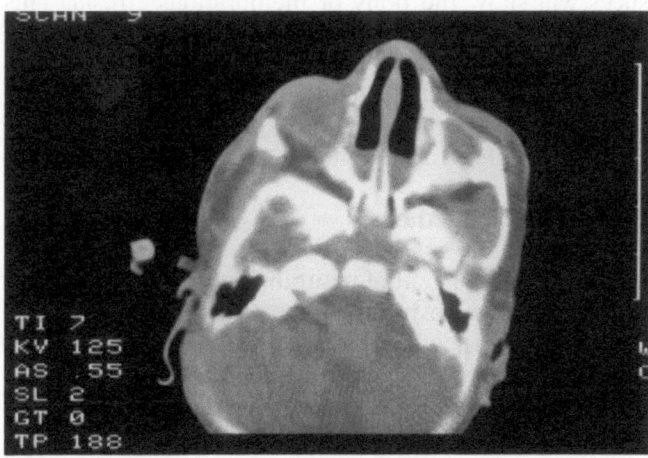

Fig. 1. Bilateral choanal atresia: note fluid levels in the nasal cavity due to bony bars causing obstruction

Table 1. Causes of upper airways tract obstruction

Neonate	Choanal atresia		
	Congenital nasopharyngel tumours		
	Trans-sphenoidal encephaloceles		
	Malformations, e.g. Pierre Robin or micrognathia		
	Laryngeal haemangioma		
	Vocal cord paralysis		
	Tracheomalacia		
	Vascular rings		
	Lymphangioma and haemangioma		
	Duplication anomalies		
Infant-Toddler	As above plus		
	Infection:	Epiglottitis	
		Laryngotracheobronchitis	
		(Diphtheria)	
		(Polio)	
		Tonsillar and adenoidal enlargement	
	Tumours:	Nasopharyngeal	Rhabdomyosarcoma
			Lymphoma
			Cervical neuroblastoma
			Haemangioma/Lymphangioma
			Mediastinal tumours
			Fibromatosis
	Trauma:	Foreign body inhalation	
		Direct neck injury	
	Loss of central drive		
Older	Tumor:	Rhabdomyosarcoma	
		Lymphoma	
		Carcinoma	
		Juvenile angiofibroma	
		Mediastinal tumors	
	Infection:	As above for infant – toddler	
		Sinus disease	
	Trauma:	As above for infant – toddler	
	Chronic hypoxia:	Pickwickian syndrome	
		Ondine's curse	

struction, the contrast remains pooled in the back of the nostril at the level of the obstruction. This is best demonstrated on a decubitus film with the infant's head lying flat on the table and chin tilted upwards. This technique has now been replaced by CT (Fig. 1). Axial CT using fine slices will show the bony or membranous atresia. This should be done following suction of the nasal cavities.

Choanal atresia may be an isolated anomaly but 60-70% of cases are associated with other congenital defects. It is a constituent feature of CHARGE association (see Table 2 for definition).

Congenital Nasal Masses

Though rare, congenital nasal masses may cause symptoms of airways obstruction by preventing nasal breathing. The incidence of such masses is said to be 1 in 20-40 000 live births. Most of the congenital nasal masses are externally visible, e.g. nasal dermoids. The most frequent congenital nasal masses leading to obstructive airways symptoms in children are the nasal meningo-encephaloceles. These are local herniations of glial tissue through a defect in the skull (Fig. 2). The nasal hernia-

tions are described as being fronto-ethmoid, naso-frontal, naso-ethmoidal or naso-orbital.

Children with such lesions may present at any age during childhood with breathing difficulties, symptoms occurring when the encephalocele obstructs the nasopharynx. Symptoms are often accentuated during feeding. Clinically, externally, there may be hypertelorism. Most are discovered by finding a mass in the infant's mouth which can vary in size depending on the amount of cerebro-spinal fluid (CSF). Once suspected, the infant requires MR imaging both to confirm the diagnosis, and to assess the presence of any associated brain anomaly, and to identify the presence of brain within the mass, although most are filled with CSF.

Table 2. Charge

C	Colobomas
H	Heart disease
A	Choanal atresia
R	Growth retardation and developmental delay
G	Genital hypoplasia in males
E	Ear deformities and deafness

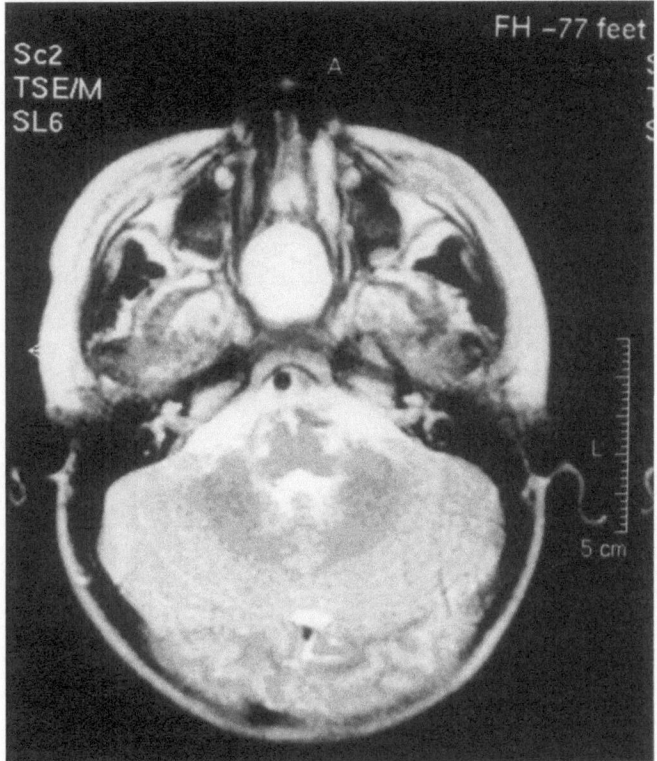

Fig. 2. Congenital midline fronto-ethmoid meningocele. T2 weighted images. The infant presented with symptoms of difficulty with breathing during eating

A rare congenital midline defect is a persistent hypophyseal canal in which the pituitary gland protrudes into the nasopharynx and appears as a "polyp". Radiographically the canal lies below the sphenoid synchondrosis and must not be confused with this.

Other Congenital Nasal Masses

These are even rarer than the rare meningoencephaloceles and include nasolacrimal duct, mucoceles, nasal hamartomas, and haemangiomas.

Craniofacial Malformations

Obstruction to breathing occurs in children with micrognathia by the tongue being too large for the small oral cavity. Similar problems with the tongue also occur in syndromes with organomegaly such as Beckwith-Wiedemann syndrome. Micrognathia occurs in many syndromes and includes craniofacial microsomia, Treacher-Collins syndrome and Pierre Robin. Maxillary hypoplasia may also lead to symptoms of airways obstruction and is a feature of some of the craniosynostosis syndromes.

The degree of airways obstruction varies. Some children will require tracheostomy. Others can be managed medically but precipitated into problems by infection. Imaging the craniofacial malformation is required when surgical in-

tervention is being planned and primarily requires CT with 3D reconstruction. Videofluoroscopy of contrast swallows may be needed to assess feeding difficulties.

Angiomatous and Lymphangiomatous Malformations

Facial cavernous and mixed haemangiomas may present at birth with a tumour mass, the mass usually growing slowly. Arteriovenous masses are rarer and grow more rapidly. These lesions cause airways obstruction either by external distortion of the airways, e.g. mouth and nose, or when they extend internally, by direct compression of the airways.

Lymphangiomas are usually multiloculated. They may be purely cystic as in a cystic hygroma, or be a mixed lymphangio-haemangioma. These fluctuate in size but may enlarge rapidly if there is bleeding into the lesion. Airways obstruction is caused by compression.

Imaging of these lesions is by ultrasound with full mapping by MR. Therapeutic radiological intervention by aspiration of the cysts and injection of sclerosing agents is one treatment option. This must always be done following full discussion with the surgical team which is responsible for the child is care.

Sinusitis, Rhinitis and Nasal Polyps

Rhinitis is most frequently due to inhaled allergens and pollutants; infective rhinitis is rare, acute bacterial sinusitis is common. Airways obstruction occurs due to accompanying blockage of the nasal airways by secretions but is usually transient, responds to medical management and seldom needs imaging. Severe rhinitis or sinus disease can lead to disruption of sleep, feeding and growth. This is most pronounced in infants and young children due to the smaller size of their airways. Older children may also suffer sleep disturbance with apnoea, especially if there is associated adenoidal enlargement.

Radiologically, the finding of mucosal thickening in the maxillary antra is a manifestation of allergic rhinosinusitis. Antral opacity can occur with acute or chronic infection, but correlates poorly with symptoms.

Complications of chronic sinusitis include the development of a mucocele which may lead to further airways obstruction by central expansion and obstruction of the nasal cavity. They may also cause proptosis. Other complications include maxillary osteomyelitis and cavernous sinus thrombosis.

Nasal polyps or cloanal polyps produce symptoms of airways obstruction as they obstruct the normal air flow. Full imaging of the extent of the disease requires CT or MR, depending on which is the most easily available.

Infection

Acute infective tonsillitis is a common childhood complaint but does not usually lead to airways obstruction.

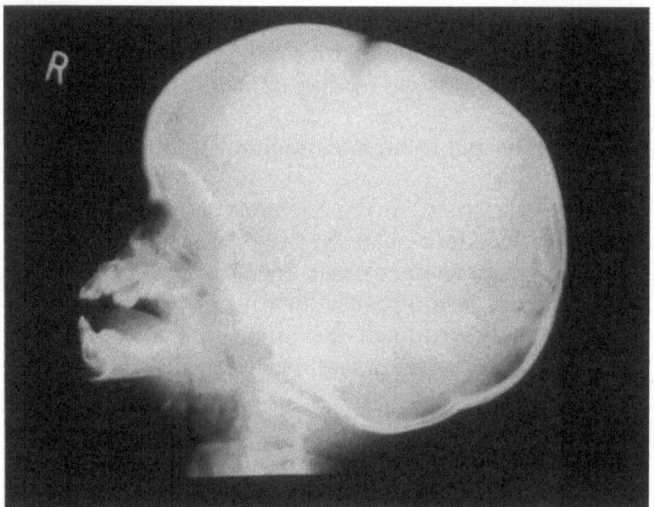

Fig. 3. Enlarged tonsils and adenoids. Note almost complete obstruction of the upper airway

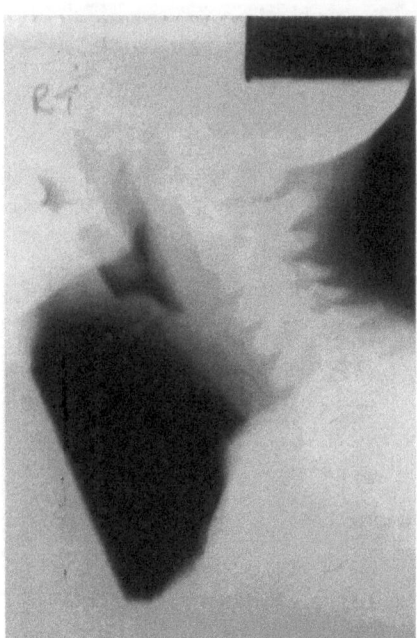

Fig. 4. Typical appearance of acute epiglottitis

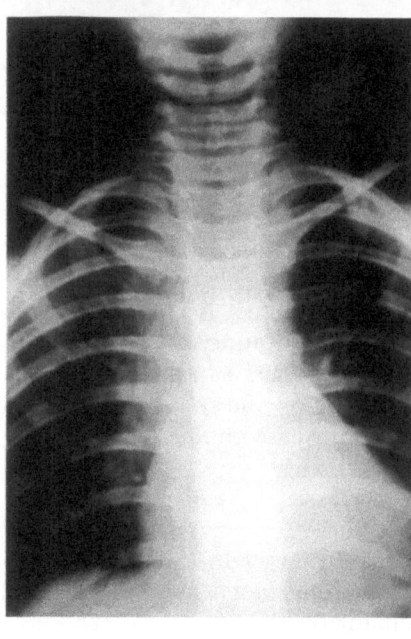

Fig. 5. Croup. Note the narrowing of the proximal trachea

Complications of acute tonsillitis that may present with symptoms of airways obstruction are quinsy or peritonsillar abscess – now rare, and a retropharyngeal abscess secondary to rupture of a retropharyngeal node.

Diphtheria is now unknown in Western society. Chronically enlarged tonsils and adenoids also cause chronic airways obstruction with snoring, sleep disturbance and consequent inattention disorders during the day (Fig. 3).

Acute Epiglottitis

Haemophilus influenza B infection is the cause of the vast majority of acute epiglottic infection. There is acute swelling of the epiglottis with usually a rapid onset of inspiratory stridor, and drooling at the mouth. The child sits upright, is pale and very distressed. It is generally agreed that radiology is not indicated and may be dangerous, as, if the child obstructs in the radiology department, resuscitation facilities may be inadequate. If in a less acute presentation, a lateral neck X-ray is taken, the epiglottis is seen to be swollen (Fig. 4).

Laryngotracheobronchitis-croup

The main infecting organisms in croup are the parainfluenza viruses, with respiratory synctial virus and rhinovirus also responsible. The infection produces inflammation of the vocal cords, but the main infection centres on the subglottic region where there is oedema, and on direct inspection ulceration may be found. In severe cases this progresses further down the trachea and bronchial tree. Hospital admission with croup is about 40 times more frequent than with acute epiglottitis.

The diagnosis of croup is usually clinically obvious and there is no need for radiology. A chest X-ray is often done because of the pyrexia. On an AP chest, if the upper airways is included in the view, a narrowing of the airway in the subglottic region is noted (Fig. 5). This has been likened to the appearance of a church steeple, on the AP view There may be associated ballooning of the hypopharynx. This occurs in both the AP and lateral view. There is frequently generalised increased bronchovascular marking within the lung fields reflecting the infection.

Retropharyngeal Abscess

This occurs most frequently by rupture of an infected retropharyngeal node, with the second most frequent

Table 3. Causes of retropharyngeal abscess

Post-perforation of a retropharyngel lymph node
Post-perforation by a foreign body
Non-accidental injury
Tuberculosis
Osteomyelitis

cause in Western society being perforation by a foreign body (Table 3). This may be accidental, iatrogenic or non-accidental. The child presents with symptoms of mouth drooling and airways obstruction.

A lateral view of the neck show loss of the normal cervical lordosis with thickening of the retropharyngeal tissues, sometimes an air fluid level, and anterior displacement of the trachea. With a typical clinical and radiological picture, further imaging is not required. If there is any suspicion of associated cervical spine osteomyelitis, then cross-sectional imaging with contrast is indicated.

Foreign Body Inhalation

Symptoms in relation to foreign body inhalation are related to the level of the obstruction. Upper airways obstruction by a foreign body can be and usually is fatal without time for radiographic intervention. A foreign body such as a piece of glass or a sweet may cause partial airways obstruction if lodged in the trachea with air passing around it. A cough or sudden movement may dislodge it so that it lies transversely and lead to sudden total obstruction.

Radiological investigation of a suspected inhaled foreign body is, by definition, only undertaken when there is a history and symptoms. An inspiratory and expiratory pair of chest X-rays are traditionally taken. In the case of upper airways signs there should be an AP and lateral view of the neck if the foreign body is likely to be opaque. With non-opaque foreign bodies the lateral view of the airways is still helpful as the foreign body may be visible.

Trauma

Trauma rarely leads to symptoms of upper airways obstruction and in most situations the cause is obvious. Inhalation and impaction, or retropharyngeal abscess due to perforation by a foreign body have already been described. Direct external neck trauma is rare but occurs during strangulation. Swelling from subcutaneous emphysema rarely causes such extensive soft tissue swelling that airway compression occurs. There is no role for neck radiology in strangulation unless it is likely to be associated with cervical spine injury, when MR is the technique of choice to exclude cord trauma. CT is required to identify the extent of the bony injury.

Subcutaneous emphysema is easy to see radiologically but when it is extensive it is impossible to see the airway properly due to the artefacts created by air in the soft tissue planes. If airway imaging is indicated, this should be done by cross-sectional imaging.

Laryngeal Causes of Airway Obstruction

Laryngomalacia

This is the commonest cause of congenital stridor. The sex incidence is equal. The stridor is inspiratory, may be intermittent and occurs during feeding or crying or when the child is asleep. Diagnosis is made by laryngoscopy.

Vocal Cord Paralysis

Vocal cord paralysis accounts for 6-13% of all causes of congenital "stridor". The diagnosis is usually made at endoscopy. Ultrasound of the vocal cords will show the paralysis.

Subglottic Stenosis

This may be congenital or acquired. The cricoid cartilage is thickened and oval in shape with thickening of the submucosa. Symptoms vary – often becoming acute when the child develops an infection. Acquired subglottic stenosis is usually a complication of intubation (Fig. 6).

Radiographs of the upper airways may show the lesion but are not reliable. Digital radiographs or CT scout films improve the visualisation but the diagnosis is one principally made at endoscopy.

Subglottic Haemangioma

Like haemangiomas elsewhere, these are hamartomas of blood vessel origin. The subglottic region is a well recognised location. The child presents with inspiratory or biphasic stridor, dyspnoea and a loud cry. Haemoptysis occurs occasionally. The diagnosis is usually endoscopic, but these lesions are also seen on ultrasound.

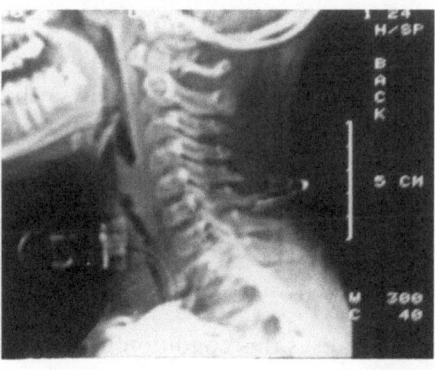

Fig. 6. Scout film for CT. Note narrowed subglottic airway; this was due to previous prolonged intubation

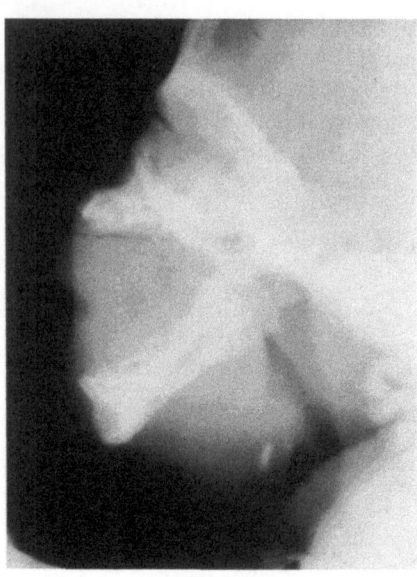

Fig. 7. Congenital teratoma causing airways obstruction due to compression and distortion of the oro and retropharyngeal airway

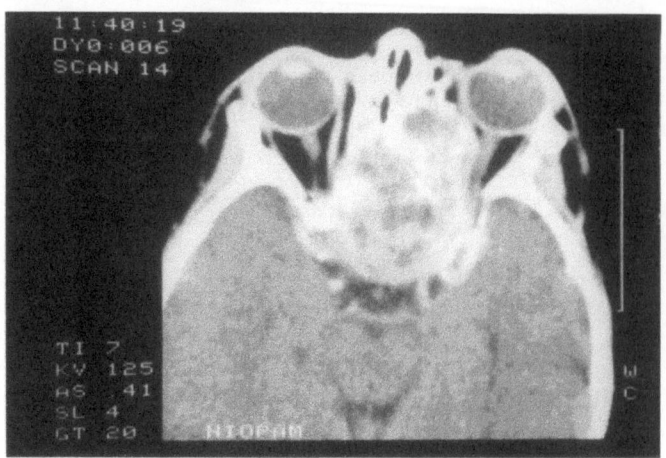

Fig. 8. Nasopharyngeal rhabdomyosarcoma. Post contrast enhanced CT. This child presented with symptoms of nasal obstruction, mouth breathing and distress when eating

Tracheomalacia

This may occur in both localised and generalised forms. The stridor of tracheomalacia is high pitched and expiratory. Cough – which is harsh and barking, is common in the localised forms. The trachea is compressed in the AP diameter with flattening of the anterior cartilaginous rings. In severe cases the two walls may appose in expiration. Some degree of tracheomalacia is almost invariable in children with oesophageal atresia and they may require aortopexy to relieve it. Tracheomalacia is also frequent in children with Down's syndrome and, as a consequence, they may be very difficult to wean from a ventilator.

Vascular Rings

Embryological maldevelopment of the origin of the great vessels may cause symptoms of airways obstruction due to tracheal compression in the mediastinum and does not fall within the remit of this chapter. The trachea may be compressed on both sides as with a double aortic arch, anteriorly most commonly by an anomalous innominate artery and posterior compression by an aberrant subclavia. This latter is not associated with airways symptoms.

Tumors

Tumors may cause symptoms of upper airways obstruction either by obstruction of the airways by infiltration or by compression and displacement of the airways. Primary neoplasms of the airways in children are rare (Fig. 7).

Laryngeal papillomatosis

The infecting agent that causes this condition is the human papilloma virus, possibly transmitted at the time of delivery. Most children present before 4 years of age. The initial symptoms are hoarseness with increasing stridor and respiratory obstruction. The papillomas start initially on the vocal cords but then progress into the upper trachea and oesophagus. They can extend into the bronchi. They may also extend to involve the nose and palate. The diagnosis is usually made by endoscopy. Narrowing of the airways may be seen in the plain radiographs. They are seen as filling defects on an oesophagogram.

Nasopharyngeal Tumors

The two most frequent tumors in this area are rhabdomyosarcomas and lymphomas, which may lead to airways obstruction [8]. The initial symptoms are variable and include pain, difficulty in feeding, blocked nose, and palpable neck nodes. Involvement of the orbits and retroorbital tissues will cause proptosis and diplopia if there is involvement of the orbital muscles.

Though bone destruction is sometimes visible on radiographs, this needs to be extensive before it is easily seen. Investigation is primarily by cross-sectional imaging. MR shows the soft tissue component to the best advantage and it also shows dural invasion. Bone destruction is easier to appreciate on CT. Though either condition can cause bone destruction, this is more frequent and more extensive with a rhabdosarcoma and nodal disease with lymphoma. The lymphoma is usually a Burkitt's lymphoma and carries a good prognosis. Nasopharyngeal rhabdosarcomas carry a very poor prognosis.

Nasopharyngeal carcinomas also occur in children and have a better prognosis than in adults. They cannot be distinguished radiologically from other nasopharyngeal tumors.

Neck Tumors

Tumors in the neck or at the thoracic inlet cause symptoms by compressing and displacing the airway. In the neck the most frequent malignant lesion by far is lymphoma. The second most frequent is a cervical neuroblastoma. This latter may present with a Horner's syndrome. If the child is X-rayed with the chin held in flexion, these lesions are easily missed. Calcification may be visible on the radiographs but this is less frequent than with abdominal masses. Full assessment is by MR and radionuclide imaging. Primitive neuroectodermal tumors also occur in the neck but cannot be distinguished from neuroblastoma without histology.

Thyroid masses are rare in children compared with the adult population. Most children present with symptoms of dysphagia or simply a palpable lump rather than airways obstruction.

A rare cause of upper airways obstruction is fibromatosis. This lesion can arise anywhere in the body. When it occurs in the neck or mediastinum, the dense fibromatous tissue may encircle the airway and cause constriction.

Conclusion

It can be seen from this outline that the potential causes of upper airways obstruction are legion. A careful history and clinical examination will usually localise the level of the obstruction so that imaging where appropriate may be tailored to identifying and mapping the causative lesion. The most frequent cause of semi-acute obstruction is infection and this is usually clinically obvious. Most of the other causes are rare and, unless one is working in a tertiary referral paediatric hospital, will seldom be encountered.

Suggested Reading

Aguado LA, Pinero BP, Betancor L, Mendez A, Banales EC (1991) Acyclovir in the treatment of laryngeal papillomatosis. Int J Pediatr Otorhinolaryngol 21: 269-274

Altmann A, Nolan T (1995) Non-intentional asphyxiation deaths due to upper airway interference in children 0 to 14 years. Inj Prev 1: 76-80

Anavi Y, Kaplinsky C, Calderon S, Zaizov R (1990) Head, neck and maxillofacial childhood Burkitt's lymphoma. A retrospective analysis of 31 patients. J Oral Maxillofac Surg 48: 708-713

Anderson GJ, Tom LWC, Womer RB, Handler SD, Wetmore RF, Potsic WP (1990) Rhabdomyosarcoma of the head and neck in children. Arch Otolaryngol Head Neck Surg 116: 428-431

Arruda LK, Mimica IM, Sole D, Weckx LL, Schoettler J, Heiner DC, et al. (1990) Abnormal maxillary sinus radiographs in children: do they represent bacterial infection? Pediatrics 85: 553-558

Cohen LM, Koltai PJ, Scott JR (1992) Lateral cervical radiographs and adenoid size: do they correlate? Ear Nose Throat J 71: 638-642

Delorimer AA, Harrison MR, Hardy K, Howell LJ, Adzick NS (1990) Tracheobronchial obstructions in infants and children. Experience with 45 cases. Ann Surg 212: 277-289

Derkay CS, Grundfast KM (1990) Airway compromise from nasal obstruction in neonates and infants. Int J Pediatr Otorhinolaryngol 19: 241-249

Emery PJ, Fearon B (1984) Vocal cord palsy in pediatric practice: a review of 71 cases. Int J Pediatr Otorhinolaryngol 8: 147-154

Garcia DP, Corbett ML, Eberly SM, Joyce MR, Le HT, Karibo JM, et al. (1994) Radiographic imaging studies in pediatric chronic sinusitis. J Allergy Clin Immunol 94: 523-530

Garel C, Contencin P, Polonovski JM, Hassan M, Narcy P (1992) Laryngeal ultrasonography in infants and children: a new way of investigating. Normal and pathological findings. Int J Pediatr Otorhinolaryngol 23: 107-115

Garel C, Hassan M, Hertz-Pannier L, Francois M, Contencin P, Narch P (1992) Contribution of MR in the diagnosis of "occult" posterior laryngeal cleft. Int J Pediatr Otorhinolaryngol 24: 177-181

Garel C, Hassan M, Legrand I, Elmaleh M, Narcy P (1991) Laryngeal ultrasonography in infants and children: pathological findings. Pediatr Radiol 21: 164-167

Heaf DP, Helms PJ, Dinwiddie R, Matthew DJ (1982) Nasopharyngeal airways in Pierre Robin syndrome. J Pediatr 100: 698-703

Irving RM, Broadbent V, Jones NS (1994) Langerhans cell histiocytosis of childhood, management of head and neck manifestations. Laryngoscope 104: 64-70

Jordan RB, Gauderer MWL (1988) Cervical teratomas: an analysis. Literature review and proposed classification. J Pediatr Surg 23: 583-591

Kaplan LC (1985) Choanal atresia and its associated anomalies. Further support for the CHARGE association. Int J Pediatr Otorhinolaryngol 8: 237-242

Myer CM III, Auringer ST, Wiatrak BJ, Bisset G (1990) Magnetic resonance imaging in the diagnosis of innominate artery compression of the trachea. Arch Otolaryngol Head Neck Surg 116: 314-316

Naegele RF, Champion J, Murphy S, Henle G, Henle W (1982) Nasopharyngeal carcinoma in American children, Epstein-Barr virus specific antibody titers and prognosis. Int J Cancer 29: 209-212

Phelps PD (1997) Radiology in paediatric otolaryngology. In: Kerr AG (ed) Scott-Brown's otolaryngology, Vol 6, 6th edn. Butterworth-Heinemann, Oxford, pp 1-24

Premachandra DJ, Milton CM (1991) Childhood haemangiomas of the head and neck. Clin Otolaryngol 16: 117-123

Ryan CA, Yacoub W, Paton T, Avard D (1990) Childhood deaths from toy balloons, paediatric intensive care unit, University of Alberta Hospitals, Edmonton, Canada. Am J Dis Child 144: 1221-1224

Singer JI, McCabe JB (1988) Epiglottitis at the extremes of age. J Emerg Med 6: 228-231

Stoohs R, Guilleminault C (1990) Obstructive sleep apnoea syndrome or abnormal upper airways resistance during sleep. J Clin Neurophysiol 7: 83-92

Imaging of Pediatric Diseases of the Tracheobronchial Tree

M. Katz,[1] E. Konen[2]

[1] Diagnostic Imaging Department, Rabin Medical Center, Campus Golda/Hasharon, Petach-Tiqwa, Israel
[2] Diagnostic Imaging Division, Tel Hashomer, Ramat Gan, Israel

Introduction

The major function of the tracheobronchial tree is to carry air to the pulmonary parenchyma and to return the modified air back to the outside. Most diseases of the trachea and bronchi come to attention because they interfere with this flow of air.

Children with disorders involving the trachea may be asymptomatic or have nonspecific symptoms (e.g. cough, dyspnea, stridor, or wheezing).

Imaging Modalities

Imaging of the pediatric trachea includes techniques that exploit almost every aspect of imaging modality available to the radiologist.

Chest X-ray

The chest radiograph (posterior-anterior and lateral) is usually the first radiographic study in patients with suspected tracheal abnormality. The high-kV (130-150 kV) frontal airway view with added filtration provides additional intrinsic contrast of the tracheobronchial tree against the adjacent mediastinal structures.

Fluoroscopy

Fluoroscopy represents a non-invasive dynamic method of evaluation of the trachea during respiratory phases (enlarges during inspiration and becomes narrow during expiration) and of anomalies such as tracheomalacia and intraluminal foreign bodies (air trapping, mediastinal shift and diaphragmatic motions are evaluated).

Barium study

Barium study of the esophagus helps in the diagnosis of congenital anomalies which affect the tracheobronchial tree, such as esophageal atresia and tracheoesophageal fistulas. It can detect extrinsic compression due to vascular rings or mediastinal masses. The choice of contrast agent and the examination technique are chosen with regard to the suspected pathology.

Tracheobronchography

Spiral computed tomography (CT) examination has almost eliminated the need for bronchography. It is still a helpful technique in the imaging of some congenital and acquired tracheobronchial anomalies in infants and children whose condition is critical and who cannot be transported; as an adjuvant step before bronchoscopy performed under fluoroscopic control; and in conditions for which dynamic assessment of the tracheobronchial tree is necessary (tracheobronchomalacia). There is -currently no approved contrast agent for this examination. The suggested contrast agents are diluted barium sulfate and non-ionic low osmolar agents (Iopamiro 300).

Angiography

Angiography is an invasive examination rarely used in the evaluation of the tracheobronchial tree in children, having been replaced by other noninvasive imaging modalities such as CT and magnetic resonance imaging (MRI). If performed, angiography has an essential role in the diagnosis and especially in the treatment of vascular anomalies (sequestration and pulmonary arteriovenous fistulas).

Magnetic Resonance Imaging

Magnetic resonance imaging (MRI) and magnetic resonance angiography (MRA) is the imaging modality that evaluates directly the trachea/bronchi and the adjacent mediastinal structures from different orientations without ionizing radiation or contrast agent injection. But an MRI examination is still more expensive, less available and of longer duration than CT examination, requiring in many instances longer periods ot anesthesia than other imaging modalities.

Computed Tomography

Computed tomography is a noninvasive imaging modality that displays the transaxial anatomy of the tracheobronchial tree and the adjacent mediastinal structures with precision and in detail. In addition on axial scans, information on the lung parenchyma and the chest wall is received without additional radiation exposure and without the overlying effect of other anatomical structures. Intrinsic or extrinsic involvement of the airway in children is readily diagnosed by CT.

Collimation, table increment and sedation/anesthesia protocols vary with the age, size of the patient, area of interest and clinical indication for examination.

Spiral/Helical CT

Spiral CT has a number of advantages over conventional CT in the examination of pediatric patients: it is more rapid, significantly decreases motion artifacts; the data can be reconstructed retrospectively without increasing radiation exposure to the child and; if contrast study is required, it can be performed during peak vascular enhancement. Being a rapid examination it decreases motion artifacts, even when scans are performed without suspended respiration and allows good contrast enhancement of vascular structures (Figs. 1a, b and 3a). Finally, high-quality two-and three-dimensional image reconstructions generated from the volumetric spiral CT

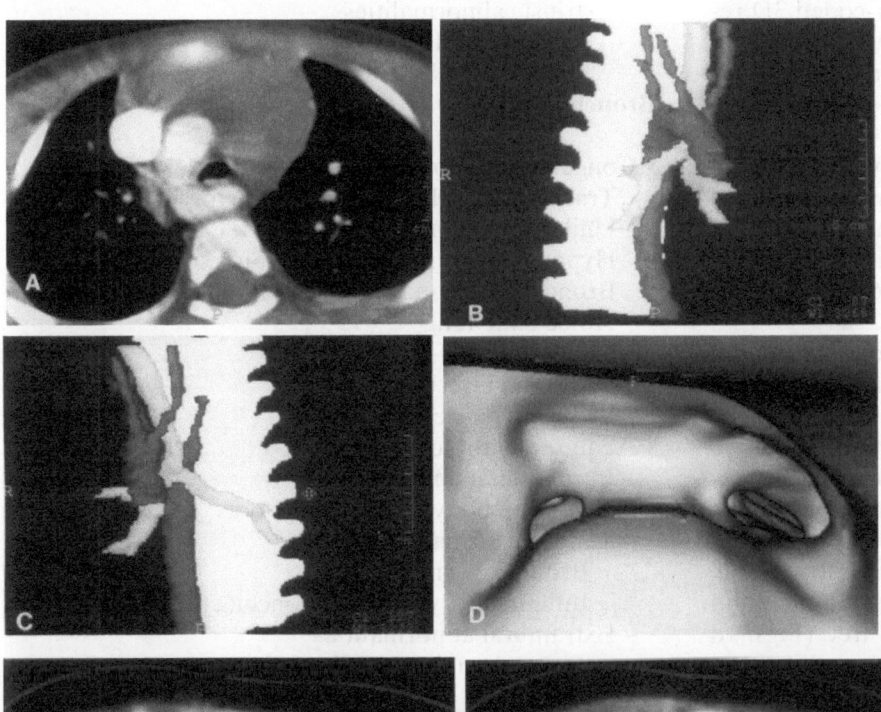

Fig. 1. a Axial image of a 2-year-old girl with a right aortic arch and left aberrant subclavian artery compressing the carinal area from behind. **b, c** Surface-shaded 3D reconstruction of the spine (*in white*), tracheo-bronchial tree (*light gray*) and aorta and its branches (*deep gray*) in right and left oblique positions. **d** Virtual bronchoscopy image at the carinal level showing a bulge on the posterior wall produced by the aberrant subclavian artery

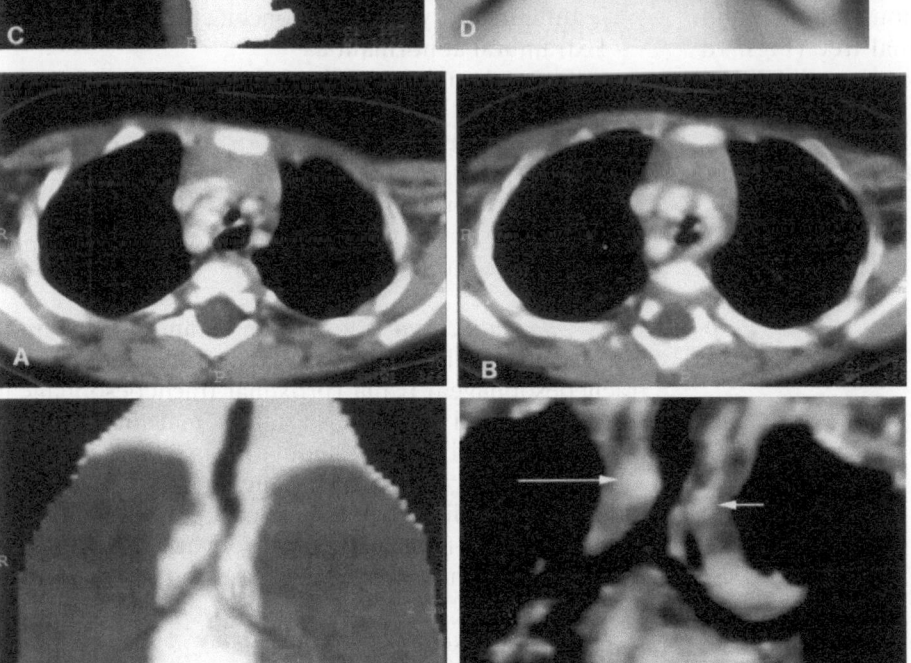

Fig. 2. a, b Axial images in an 8-month-old boy (following contrast injection) with complete double aortic arch at different levels. **c** Minimum intensity projection (minIP). **d** Multiplanar reconstruction of the airways show vascular compressions (by two complete different aortic arches) on both sides of the trachea (*arrows*)

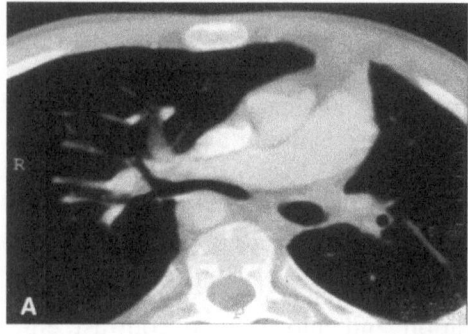 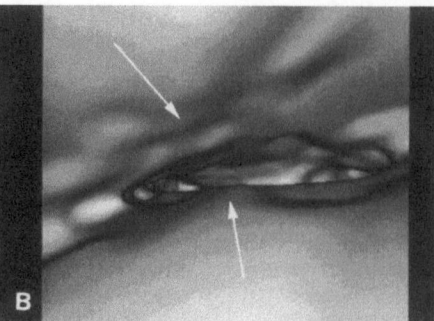

Fig. 3. a Axial image in a 12-year-old boy with absent left pulmonary artery and left hypoplastic lung and compression of right main bronchus between the right main bronchus and the right descending aorta. **b** Virtual bronchoscopy image at the carina shows the extrinsic compression on the origin of the right main bronchus (*arrows*)

data can be obtained. There are three main rendering techniques available to date on spiral CT:

- *Shaded surface display* as grey or color-coded 3D reconstruction that depicts complex anatomic relationships, particularly in regions of overlapping structures (Fig. 1b and c).
- *Maximum intensity projection* which permits good separation of the enhanced lumen of vascular structures and gives images as informative as angiographic studies. On the other hand minimum intensity projection (minIP) displays air-containing structures giving information on the tracheobronchial tree and the pulmonary parenchyma (Fig. 2c).
- *Curved planar reformation* uses curved or angulated planes of section for optimal detection of structures with a non-linear configuration.

Virtual bronchoscopy represents a new noninvasive technique that provides an internal view of the tracheobronchial tree and is useful as a complementary study to fiberoptic bronchoscopy. The information results from postprocessing of the axial images on a separate console and permits simultaneous visualization of inner and outer structures of the tracheobronchial tree (Figs. 1d and 3b).

Classification of Tracheobronchial Pathology in Children

Trachea

- Congenital malformations
    Esophageal atresia
    Tracheoesophageal fistula
    Tracheal agenesis
    Vascular rings (Figs. 1 and 2)
- Acquired pathology
  - Intraluminal abnormalities
      Foreign bodies
  - Mural abnormalities
      Papillomatosis
      Hemangiomas
      Membranous croup
      Congenital/acquired tracheal stenosis

    Tracheomalacia (isolated/associated)
    Tracheobronchomegaly
  - Extrinsic abnormalities
      Tumor/lymphoma

Bronchi

- Congenital malformations
    Tracheal bronchus/ cardiac bronchus
    Unilateral pulmonary agenesis
    Hypogenetic lung syndrome (Fig. 3)
    Broncho-pulmonary sequestration
    Horse-shoe lung
    Isomerism
    Bronchial atresia
    Bronchogenic cyst
- Acquired pathology
  - Intraluminal abnormalities
      Foreign body
  - Mural abnormalities
      Bronchial tumor
      Inflammatory process/bronchiectasis
  - Extramural abnormalities
      Tumor/lymphoma/enlarged heart/enlarged pulmonary arteries
  - Postoperative pathology
      Transplanted lung
      Tracheal/bronchial stents
  - Trauma
      Tracheal/bronchial rupture

Esophageal atresia is a relative common congenital anomaly and in the majority of cases is associated with a tracheoesophageal fisula (proximal tracheoesophageal fistula 1%, distal fistula 82-86%, proximal and distal fistula 1%, isolated fistula without atresia 6%).

The diagnosis (clinical and radiologic) is made during the first days of life except in the case of an isolated tracheoesophageal fistula, which is brought to attention by recurrent pneumonias or by an increased amount of intestinal gas.

Tracheal agenesis is a rare anomaly. The whole or a part of the trachea is absent. The lungs are aerated through a narrow connection of the tracheal bifurcation area to the esophagus. The condition is suspected immediately after birth when there is severe respiratory distress, and can be confirmed by tracheobronchography.

Vascular rings represent a group of congenital anomalies in which the trachea and the esophagus are encircled by the aortic arch and its branches. A vascular ring may be incomplete and rarely presents with symptoms. If the vascular ring is complete the symptoms are usually due to tracheal compression, such as wheezing or respiratory distress. Esophageal symptoms are rare and less dramatic.

There are different patterns of vascular rings: a) symptomatic: double aortic arch, right aortic arch with left aberrant subclavian artery, aberrant left pulmonary artery (Figs. 1 and 2); b) occasionally or usually asymptomatic: left aortic arch with left aberrant subclavian artery, left aortic arch with right descending aorta, anomalous innominate artery.

Since the esophagus represents the "sentinel" of the trachea in the diagnosis of compression by vascular rings, the first examinations required are chest X-ray and barium esophagram. Further preoperative assessment is performed either by MRI or by CT examination. The role of different reconstruction techniques developed in the last few years is increasing and they give the surgeons a better spatial orientation before the repair procedure.

Foreign bodies, seldom located in the trachea, are recognized (if opaque) on chest X-ray by their position with the long diameter in anterior posterior projection.

Subglottic hemangiomas and papillomas are rare in children. They present with stridor; some of them regress spontaneously.

Tracheomalacia is a condition in which a segment of trachea collapses 50% or more of its maximal cross-sectional area. There are cases of primary tracheomalacia, but in the majority of patients this condition is recognized in association with or after treatment for esophageal atresia, tracheoesophageal fistula, vascular ring, longstanding intubation or bronchopulmonary dysplasia. Fluoroscopy and tracheobronchography have an important role in the imaging of this condition prior to fiberoptic bronchoscopy.

Congenital *tracheal stenosis*, isolated or in conjunction with other anomalies occurs when the membranous portion of the trachea is absent or nearly absent and the tracheal wall consists of complete cartilaginous rings. The outcome of this entity is variable from progressive respiratory distress to death; rare cases are able to survive without surgery due to tracheal cartilage growth. It is of great importance to determine the length, degree and severity of the stenotic segment of the trachea, bifurcation and main-stem bronchi.

Diagnostic imaging has an important role since it is usually the only way to provide this information since many stenoses are too narrow to permit the passage of a bronchoscope. High KV frontal airway view and tracheobronchography are used for the diagnosis of this entity. Today spiral CT and its 3D reconstruction are beginning to represent an alternative method of diagnosis.

The involvement of the trachea by *extrinsic lesions* (mediastinal tumors or lymphomas) comes to attention indirectly during different imaging procedures for diagnosis and staging of the primary lesions (chest X-ray, CT, MRI).

Tracheal bronchus represents a separate bronchus to the right upper lobe arising independently from the trachea.

Unilateral pulmonary agenesis is a rare anomaly of bronchial branching and is associated with other anomalies such as patent ductus arteriosus, ventricular septal defect, imperforate anus or tracheoesophagea fistula. The diagnosis is made initially by chest X-ray and confirmed by CT or MRI examination.

Bronchial atresia is obliteration of the lumen of segmental bonchus. It is usually minimally symptomatic; hence, no treatment is required. The condition is diagnosed by chest X-ray and CT scan examinations.

Bronchial foreign bodies represent a frequent problem in pediatric radiology. In 85% the source is of vegetable origin and the location is almost exclusively in lower lobes.

In the acute phase the radiologic manifestations are: obstructive overinflation (68%), collapse (30%), infiltrate (11%), radiopaque foreign body, air trapping (inspiratory/expiratory films, lateral decubitus films or fluoroscopy).

Bronchial tumors are rare in children.

Bronchiectasis represents localized (irreversible) dilatation of the bronchial tree. It is classified as: a) cylindrical/tubular; b) saccular/cystic; or c) varicose bronchiectasis.

The etiology is variable: congenital as in bronchial atresia, immotile cilia syndrome, abnormal secretions such as in cystic fibrosis, immunodeficiencies, allergic bronchopulmonary aspergillosis, chronic infection, repeated episodes of aspiration. Bronchography has been replaced by CT (minIP and high resolution computed tomography, HRCT) in the diagnosis of bronchiectasis.

The most frequent cause of *external/extramural bronchial compression* is represented by lymphoma. Other rare causes are: inflammatory hilar adenopathy, a dilated heart and dilated pulmonary vessels. The diagnosis is establibed by plain X-ray, CT and/or MRI.

Spiral CT examination and its different reconstruction modalities (minIP and multiplanar reconstructions) are valuable especially in *lung transplant* recipients. In these patients the major role of imaging is the recognition of airway complications, such as: dehiscence and stenosis at the anastomosis of the native and transplanted bronchi.

Tracheal/bronchial stents: in the last few years stents have been placed in patients with extensive strictures or external compressions. The position of these stents is readily identifiable on spiral CT; multiplanar reconstruction along the long axis of the airway helps to localize the exact stent position.

Rupture/fracture of the trachea/bronchus is rare in children and is accompanied by fracture of the upper ribs, pneumothorax, pneumomediastinum, subcutaneous emphysema, collapsed lung, inadequate reexpansion of lung despite chest tube insertion (due to air leak). The location of rupture is just above the carina or at the main-stem bronchus close to its origin. Since the mortality rate is high in this entity, CT examination plays an important role in the early diagnosis.

Suggested Reading

Kirks RK, Griscom NT (1998) Practical pediatric imaging, diagnostic radiology of infants and children. Lippincott-Raven, Philadelphia, pp 659-667

Griscom NT (1993) Diseases of the trachea, bronchi and smaller airways. Radiol Clin North Am 31: 605-615

Danhert W (1998) Radiology review manual. Williams & Wilkins, Baltimore, pp 229-507

Katz M, Konen E, Rozenman J, Szeinberg A, Itzchak Y (1995) Spiral CT and 3D image reconstruction of vascular rings and associated tracheobronchial anomalies. J Comput Assist Tomogr 19: 564-568

Konen E, Katz M, Rozenman J, Ben Shlush A, Itzchak Y, Szeinberg A (1998) Virtual bronchoscopy in children: early clinical experience. AJR 171: 1699-1702

Manson D, Filler R, Gordon R (1996) Tracheal growth in congenital tracheal stenosis. Pediatr Radiol 26: 427-430

Desai DP, Holinger LD, Gonzales-Crusi F (1998) Tracheal neoplasms in children. Ann Otol Rhinol Laryngol 107: 790-795

LoCicero J, Costello P, Campos CT, et al. (1996) Spiral CT with multiplanar and three-dimensional reconstructions accurately predicts tracheobronchial pathology. Ann Thorac Surg 62: 811-817

Griscom NT (1991) CT measurement of the tracheal lumen in children and adolescents. AJR 156: 371-372

Vogl T, Wilimzig C, Bilaniuk LT, et al. (1990) MR imaging in pediatric airway obstruction. J Comput Assist Tomogr 14: 182-186

Thopson IM, Whittlesey, Slovis TL, et al. (1997) Evaluation of contrast media for bronchography. Pediatr Radiol 27: 598-605

Manson D, Babyn P, Filler R, Holowka S (1994) Three-dimensional imaging of the pediatric trachea in congenital tracheal stenosis. Pediatr Radiol 24: 175-179

Lee T, Lee SK (1997) Upper airway obstruction in infants and children: evaluation by tracheobronchography with a nonionic contrast agent. Pediatr Radiol 27: 276-280

Bar-Ziv J, Solomon A (1990) Direct coronal CT scanning of tracheo-bronchial, pulmonary and thoraco-abdominal lesions in children. Pediatr Radiol 20: 245-248

Siegel M, Lucker GD (1995) Pediatric applications of helical (spiral) CT. Radiol Clin North Am 33: 997-1007

Mediastinal and Hilar Neoplasia in Children

H.G. Ringertz[1,2], M. Lidegran[2]

Department of Radiology[1] and Pediatric Radiology[2], Karolinska Hospital, Stockholm, Sweden

Introduction

Mediastinal and hilar masses in children are challenging to the radiologist but also rewarding as the diagnosis and therapeutic alternatives depend on the imaging findings. These findings have to be interpreted in the light of size, location, and relation to the other intrathoracic structures. Anatomically the mediastinum includes all intrathoracic viscera except the lungs and pleura. A useful classification of the mediastinal masses is based on dividing mediastinum in an anterior, a middle, and a posterior compartment [1] as seen in Fig. 1.

These compartments can be identified on lateral chest X-rays or on transaxial or sagittal tomographic sections with computed tomography (CT) or magnetic resonance imaging (MRI). As the size of the pediatric mediastinal or hilar masses vary considerably the differ-ential diagnostic use of the compartment refers to the centre of the mass as seen in a lateral projection. There are neoplasms like lymphoma or mesenchymal tumors that can be localised in all three compartments, but others, like teratoma and germ cell tumors in the anterior compartment, or neurogenic tumors in the posterior, only occur in one compartment.

In a recent study of pediatric chest tumors [2] 39% of the masses were mediastinal in location. Of these 63% were primary and malignant, 26% were benign and the remaining 11% metastatic. The dominating malignant diagnoses were Hodgkin's disease, non-Hodgkin's lymphoma, and neuroblastoma, all three of which were of about the same frequency. The most frequent benign diagnosis was normal thymus simulating an anterior mediastinal mass.

Mediastinal masses are by definition extrapleural and

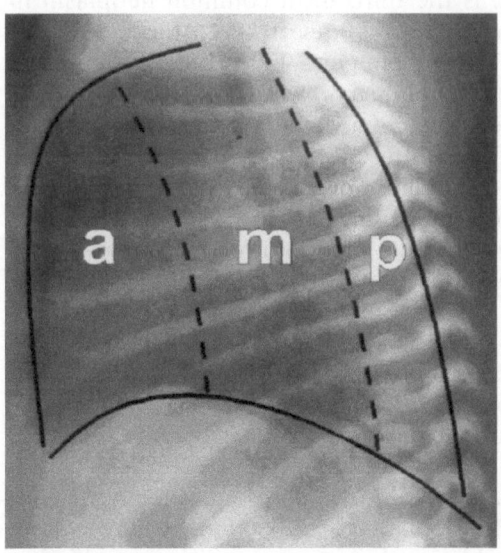

Fig. 1. Definition of anterior (a), middle (m), and posterior (p) mediastinal compartments in a neonate. The border between the middle and posterior mediastinum is defined as a curved coronal plane through the anterior margins of the vertebral bodies. The border between the anterior and middle compartment is parallel to the other through the upper tip of manubrium of sternum

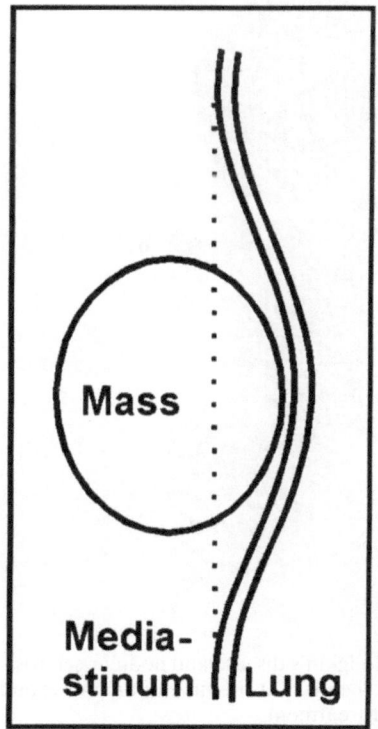

Fig. 2. Typical deformity of the medial pleural re-flection caused by a me-diastinal mass. Well de-fined, convex border to-wards the lung and sharp angles away from the mass of the cranial and caudal limits of the deformity

tend to have corresponding radiologic features. Thus, they are convex towards the lung and the cranial and caudal borders tend to have a sharp angle away from the mass as seen in Fig. 2. However, from a differential diagnostic point of view a number of pulmonary lesions that mimic mediastinal masses have to be discussed as well.

Anterior Mediastinum

Normal thymus is sometimes misdiagnosed as a mediastinal mass (Fig. 3). Most frequently this occurs with an unusually large or unusually shaped thymus in the in-

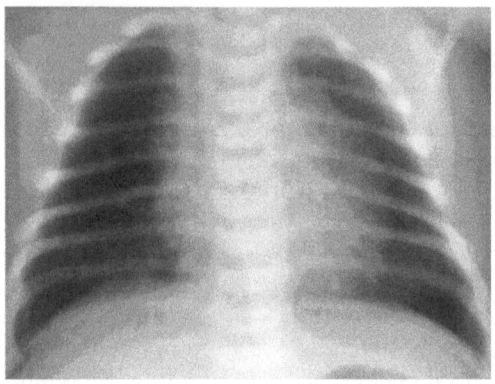

Fig. 3. Normal thymus in a young infant. The most frequent pseudotumor of the anterior mediastinum. The typical wave sign of the lateral thymic contour is one possibility to avoid the incorrect diagnosis of a neoplasm in a case like this

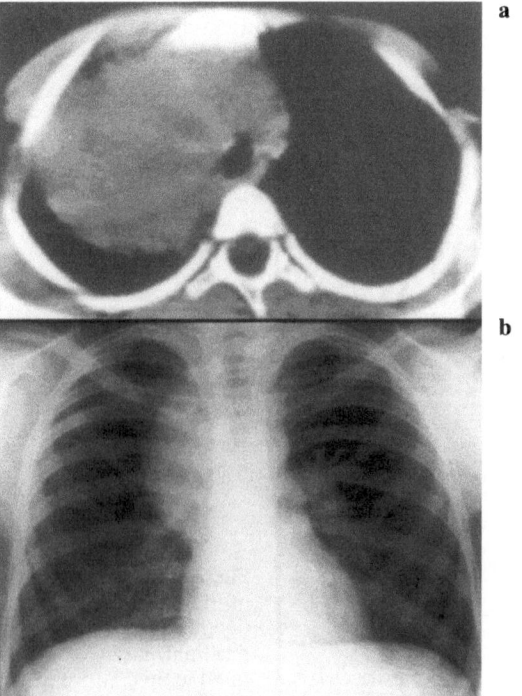

Fig. 4. Teenage boy with Hodgkin's disease and nodular sclerosis **a** on a CT section through the mass at the time of diagnosis and **b** on an AP chest film after treatment

fant or with a large thymus in the older child. Ultrasound demonstrates a homogenous echogenicity and no displacement of vascular structures. Thymic enlargement can be caused by endocrine disorders and sometimes as a reaction after chemotherapy. Ectopic thymic tissue is seen in the upper mediastinum and close to the thyroid in 20% of small children [3].

Thymoma is very rare in childhood. About two thirds grow within a capsule while the remaining infiltrate through the capsule. They are frequently associated with either paraneoplastic syndromes or myasthenia gravis [4].

Germ cell tumors originate from primitive germ cells that give rise to, e.g. seminoma and embryonic carcinoma. These cells may further differentiate into embryonic tissue causing teratoma or extraembryonic tissue to form endodermal sinus tumors and choriocarcinoma. Mixtures of these forms are called mixed germ cell tumors. Only about 3% of germ cell tumors occur in the mediastinum, mostly in the anterior part near or within the thymus. They represent one fourth of all anterior mediastinal tumors in children, less in adults. Eighty percent of all are benign and the most common type is teratoma, 65%.

Mature teratomas contain different well-developed tissue elements while immature teratomas are made up of tissues of fetal type. The latter are often benign in childhood while they are malignant in adults. The inhomogenous structure and midline position are the characteristic imaging findings of these neoplasms. With large germ cell tumors the radiological findings include bronchial compression, mediastinal adenopathy, and contralateral lung metastases.

Lymphoma is the third most common neoplasm in children and constitutes about 10%. Of those 60% are non-Hodgkin's lymphoma and 40% Hodgkin's disease. Non-Hodgkin's lymphoma may be difficult to differentiate from acute lymphocytic leukemia in pediatric imaging. However, the differences between non-Hodgkin's lymphoma and Hodgkin's disease are marked, both considering imaging appearance and response to therapy.

Residual mediastinal masses after lymphoma treatment can constitute an imaging problem. In a recent follow-up study of 24 cases of Hodgkin's disease, 10 of non-Hodgkin's lymphoma and 5 with anaplastic lymphoma the residual masses after treatment were generally benign [5]. The authors conclude that radiological follow-up is sufficient except when a treatment protocol requires surgical verification.

Non-Hodgkin's lymphoma presents mostly in children around 10 years of age, only one quarter of whom are girls. The histopathological classification, the frequency, location and cell types are seen in Table 1. The mediastinum is the second most common site in about one fourth of the cases. The mass is normally extranodal in contrast to Hodgkin's disease and adult non-Hodgkin's lymphoma.

Table 1. Histopathology of pediatric non-Hodgkin's lymphoma with frequency, location, and cell types

Non-Hodgkin's lymphoma Histopathologic classification	Frequency in childhood (%)	Location and cell types
• Non-lymphoblastic Undifferentiated		
Burkitt	20-25	Abdominal, ileocecal, derived from B-cells
Non-Burkitt	25-30	Abdominal, ileocecal, derived from B-cells
Histiocytic	15-20	Seldom mediastinal
• Lymphoblastic	30-35	Supradiaphragmatic, mediastinal mass, often cervical, derived from T-cells

Hodgkin's disease in childhood is from a histologic point of view dominated by nodular sclerosis (65%), followed by mixed cellularity, lymphocytic predominance and depletion. About 85% of children with Hodgkin's disease have mediastinal engagement, but nearly all have cervical adenopathy. Abdominal para-aortic lymph nodes and the spleen are much less involved. Hodgkin's disease normally originates in lymph nodes and in the mediastinum most frequently hilar and subcarinal nodes are enlarged (Fig. 4). Tracheo-bronchial compression, pleural effusion and infiltration of the pulmonary parenchyma are frequent imaging findings in children with Hodgkin's disease. Pulmonary infiltrates are however only seen together with hilar lymphadenopathy.

Lymphangiomas are benign tumors resulting from malformation of the lymphatic system in the mediastinum. They are rare and may occur in the anterior, middle, or posterior mediastinum in descending order of frequency. They are cystic which can be demonstrated with ultrasound, CT, or MRI [6].

Middle Mediastinum

Adenopathy can be caused by inflammatory or malignant disease. Most mediastinal lymph node locations are located in the middle mediastinum along trachea, below the bifurcation of trachea or in the pulmonary hilum around the bronchi. Adenopathy represents hard lymph nodes that can cause indentations of the adjacent airway. Low CT attenuation of the nodes is seen with necrosis due to aggressive malignant disease or infection while high attenuation can be seen with other malignant lymph node metastases. Calcification can represent tuberculosis, fungal infection or musculoskeletal tumor metastases.

Bronchopulmonary foregut malformations are formed during the critical embryogenic period of the foregut. Thus, this group includes both enteric and bronchogenic malformations. Of this large group of congenital thoracic anomalies the most frequent, that is bronchogenic cysts, the intra- and extra-lobar pulmonary sequestrations, neurenteric cysts, and enteric cysts will be discussed below.

Bronchogenic cysts can become symptomatic throughout childhood, but most frequently in the neonatal period. They may cause pulmonary airtrapping and are often located as a mass between the trachea and oesophagus. Sometimes they have a systemic blood supply and are part of the pulmonary sequestration complex. They can have communication with the gastrointestinal tract and most often the oesophagus.

Pulmonary sequestration is generally defined as "a mass of lung tissue with no normal connection with the bronchial tree or the pulmonary arteries". It is most frequently located in the lower lobes in the segments close to the diaphragm. Of the two types, intra- and extralobar sequestration, the latter is located on the left side in 9 out of 10 cases. The mass is normally diagnosed on plain film but for bronchial or vascular details MRI (MRA) and sometimes CT or even bronchography is used.

Neurenteric cysts are normally seen in either the middle or the posterior mediastinum, often together with various vertebral malformations or anomalies. They are all associated with an abnormal closure of the primitive neurenteric canal. There can be hemivertebrae, spina bifida anterior or posterior, or just scoliosis often at a level above that of the neurenteric cyst itself.

Enteric cysts in the mediastinum are most often gastrogenic and contain a gastric mucosa that produces acid and pepsin. This will often result in an early but potentially life-threatening presentation due to perforation into adjacent structures such as the bronchial tree or the pleura.

Posterior Mediastinum

Neurogenic tumors represent 29% of all mediastinal tumors in children [7] and they dominate the tumors in the posterior mediastinum. Neurofibroma and schwannoma arise from peripheral nerve and nerve sheath while ganglioneuroma, ganglioneuroblastoma and neuroblastoma arise from sympathetic ganglia. The latter group represents about 85% of these neurogenic tumors in children but only 25% in adults.

Neuroblastoma in the mediastinum normally occurs before the age of 2 years and always before 5 years and represents about 15% of all neuroblastomas. The tumor cells are entirely undifferentiated sympatoblasts and

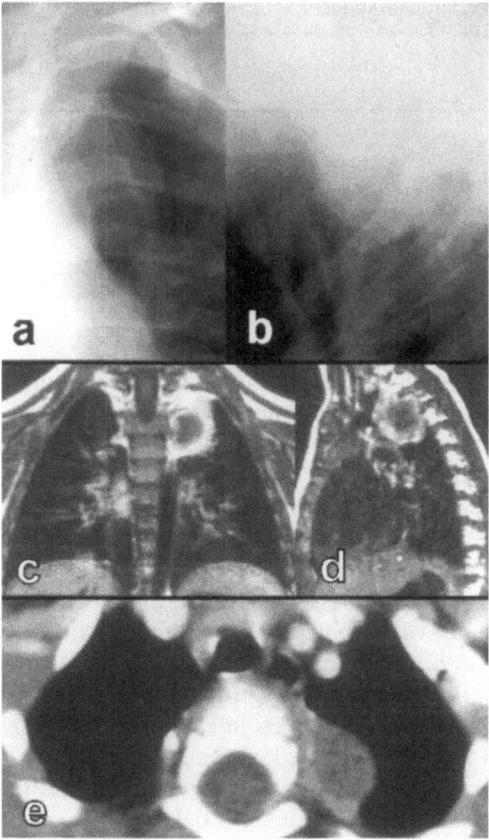

Fig. 5. Accidentally diagnosed stage 1 neuroblastoma in a two year old girl. Typical imaging findings from chest films **a** in AP and **b** lateral projection illustrating the mass location in the posterior mediastinum. T1 weighted MRI with **c** a coronal and **d** a sagittal slice through the centre of the mass demonstrate a central necrotic portion with a high intensity rim around. A CT transaxial section **e** after contrast media administration also relates the mass to the surrounding mediastinal structures.

may be difficult to differentiate from the cells of Ewing's tumor, rhabdomyosarcoma and lymphoma. Mediastinal neuroblastoma contains radiologically detectable calcifications in about 40% of cases.

The tumor is normally not diagnosed until it influences adjacent structures or metastasizes (Fig. 5). Compared to other locations mediastinal neuroblastoma demonstrates intraspinal, extradural extension more frequently. The mass is normally well seen on chest radiographs but CT and/or MRI is required to evaluate the extension of the mass. CT demonstrates soft-tissue attenuation but following contrast injection the enhancement is often inhomogenous. On both T1 and T2 weighted MRI images the tumor tends to have high signal intensity. Mediastinal neuroblastoma has a much better prognosis than abdominal neuroblastoma with a three times higher survival rate. The survival for infants below 1 year of age is five times higher than for children older than 2 years.

Ganglioneuroblastoma is more highly differentiated than neuroblastoma and a less malignant tumor that is relatively more frequent with close to 50% located in the mediastinum. Its general occurrence is, however, less frequent and the age spectrum is somewhat higher than for neuroblastoma. The imaging characteristics are the same as for its more malignant relative but these tumors have a good prognosis even after 1 year of age.

Ganglioneuroma is a mature benign tumor that occurs in older children. Histologically the tumor consists mainly of mature ganglion cells. The mass is encapsulated and often contains large calcifications.

Vascular mediastinal masses in children are most frequently aneurysms of aorta, the main pulmonary artery, the right or the left pulmonary artery. The vascular masses are most frequent in the posterior compartment of the mediastinum but can also occur in the anterior or middle.

Differential Pulmonary Lesions

A mediastinal abscess can cause a mass or a widening of the mediastinum. Such an abscess can be caused by spread from a pneumonia, from esophageal perforation, or be iatrogenic following surgery [8]. Malignant parenchymal lung tumors in children are dominated by metastatic lesions. When located close to the mediastinum direct overgrowth can occur and it can be difficult to differentiate between large metastases and mediastinal neoplasia from a radiological point of view.

References

1. Kirks DR (1998) Practical pediatric imaging. Diagnostic radiology of infants and children, 3rd edn. Lippincott-Raven, Philadelphia New York, p 777
2. Wyttenbach R, Vock P, Tschäppeler H (1998) Cross-sectional imaging with CT and/or MRI of pediatric chest tumors. Eur Radiol 8: 1040-1046
3. Leonidas JC (1998) The thymus: from past misconception to present recognition. Pediatr Radiol 28: 275-282
4. Rosado-de-Christenson ML, Galobardes J, Moran CA (1992) Thymoma: radiologic-pathologic correlation. Radiographics 12: 151-168
5. Brisse H, Pacquement H, Burdairon E, Plancher C, Neuenschwander S (1998) Outcome of residual mediastinal masses of thoracic lymphomas in children: impact on management and radiological follow-up strategy. Pediatr Radiol 28: 444-450
6. Ablin DS, Azouz EM, Jain KA (1995) Large intrathoracic tumors in children: imaging findings. AJR 165: 925-934
7. Naidich DP, Webb WR, Müller NL, Krinsky GA, Zerhouni EA, Siegelman SS (1999) Computed tomography and magnetic resonance of the thorax, 3rd edn. Lippincott-Raven, Philadelphia New York
8. Fields JM, Schwartz DS, Gosche J, Keller MS (1997) Idiopathic bilateral anterior mediastinal abscesses. Pediatr Radiol 27: 596-597

High Resolution Computed Tomography of Diffuse Pediatric Pulmonary Diseases

J.P. Kuhn

Department of Radiology, Children's Hospital of Buffalo, Buffalo, New York, USA and
State University of New York at Buffalo, School of Medicine and Biomedical Sciences, Buffalo, New York, USA

Introduction

High resolution computed tomography (HRCT) is used to maximize spatial resolution in the lung. Most authors define this technique as the combined use of images of 1-3 mm collimation and a high spatial frequency (edge-enhancing algorithm), which on many scanners is called the "bone algorithm". When used together, these two factors result in images of the lung that approximate the appearance of a gross anatomic specimen [1, 2]. Despite intense interest and experience with this technique in diseases affecting adults, there remains little information in the literature regarding application of this technique to diseases of the child's lung [3-6].

Technique

The techniques needed for optimal HRCT have been described in detail previously [7, 8], and will only be briefly summarized her.

Slice Thickness

To optimize spatial resolution, it is necessary to use a relatively thin slice; most authors use 1.5 mm collimation but successful results have also been obtained at 3 mm thickness, which is the technique we most often utilize. Murata et al. [9] have shown no diagnostic difference between 1.5 mm and 3 mm slice thickness although the images are slightly sharper using the thinner slice. Some structures, however, are more difficult to recognize using a thinner slice. For instance, branching vessels, when sliced thinly enough, are visualized as dots and are not as easily recognized as vessels.

Slice Intervals

There is no universally applicable rule for the choice of slice intervals. Decisions must be individualized depending on the size of the child's lungs and the clinical indication for the examination. If detection of metastatic disease is the clinical indication then contiguous slices of intermediate thickness are probably the best. If searching for bronchiectasis, one would choose the thinnest slice available, perhaps at 5-10 mm increments. For our general technique, we use 6 mm slices with a 2 mm gap to minimize radiation exposure but then use either 1.5 or 3.0 mm slices through an area of interest if additional detail is required. Under 1 year of age, we prefer 3 mm slices with a 1 mm gap and 1.5 mm slices to maximize detail.

Algorithm

The reconstruction algorithm is of major importance in maximizing spatial resolution. The contrast in the lung is inherently great between the air-containing lung and the normal and abnormal tissues, which are of at least water attenuation and which may be soft tissue or calcific. The use of an edge-enhancing algorithm maximizes spatial resolution at the expense of contrast resolution and results in the production of images that are inherently noisy and appear grainy; however, this appearance does not usually hamper interpretation. Most authors advocate using the algorithm that provides the highest spatial resolution.

Field of View

Using a 512^2 matrix on a 40 cm field of view results in a pixel size of 0.78 mm but if one can use a 20 cm field of view, the pixel size can be reduced to 0.49 mm. For infants, and for the ultimate in spatial resolution, one can use a 12 cm field of view and obtain a pixel size of 0.25 mm. By combining a thin-slice, spatial-enhancing algorithm and a small field of view, it is possible to see structures between 0.3 and 0.5 mm in size.

Motion

The most important factor limiting the use of chest computed tomography (CT) in children is the problem of motion. Even in patients who can breath-hold, physiologic motion is present at the cardiac margins especially in the left lower lobe. However, nothing degrades an image like a screaming infant! We have used an Imatron (San Francisco, CA; USA) electron beam (ultrafast) CT scanner for the past 10 years [3]. All of the images not otherwise identified in this paper were made on this scanner that has a routine 0.1 s scan time allowing us to perform HRCT on critically ill patients and on even the most uncooperative infants. We sedate less than 2% of our patients and even fewer for chest CT. For many radiologists, however, optimal pediatric chest CT remains limited to the older cooperative child or to those who can be sedated. The advent of helical CT has had a positive impact on examination of the pediatric chest and allows for scanning of less cooperative children but some sedation may still be necessary.

Radiation Exposure

Radiation exposure for chest CT varies with the scanner used, the kilovoltage (KV) and the milliamperage seconds (MAS) employed, the number of slices, and the extent to which the slices overlap. It has been shown that reducing the milliamperage from 400 to 40 results in the production of somewhat noisy images but there does not appear to be any loss of diagnostic information [10, 11]. The electron beam CT scanner uses a routine scan time of 0.1 s with approximately 600 milliamperage (MA) or 60 milliamperage seconds. The entrance dose to the skin of the back is approximately 500 millirads. The total dose can be further minimized by using contiguous slices only when absolutely necessary.

Normal Lung Anatomy

Attenuation of the Normal Lung

The attenuation of the normal air-containing lung varies with the phase of respiration and with the region of the lung being examined. Attenuation is lower anteriorly than posteriorly because there is more blood in the more dependent portions of the lung; therefore, attenuation is also lower in the upper lung zones than in the lower lungs. In children, the normal lung CT density averages -600 to -700 Hounsfield units (HU) which is somewhat higher than in adults (-700 to -800 HU) and tends to be higher in younger children than in older ones. There is normally about 100 to 150 HU difference between inspiration and expiration [3]. Always viewing the images at the same window and level helps to familiarize the radiologist with what is normal for each age, but in most cases, abnormalities do not involve the lung uniformly. Regions of abnormal attenuation are thus usually readily evident by comparison with other normal regions of the lung which serve as internal reference points.

Normal Lung Structure

Space does not allow for extensive review of the pertinent normal anatomy of the lung, a subject which is well covered in the literature [5, 12, 13]. However, a brief review is necessary to form a basis for understanding the normal and abnormal CT appearances. Although up to 90% of normal lung is composed of air-containing alveoli, it is important to understand the tissue structure of the lung. Weibel and colleagues [14, 15] have described the interstitial portion of the lung as being composed of axial, peripheral and septal components. The bronchi and the pulmonary arteries form the core or axial component and travel to the lung periphery in a common loose connective tissue sheath. In most regions of the lung, the bronchus and accompanying artery are normally about the same size. Abnormalities in the perivascular space whether they result from airway inflammatory disease or perivascular or peribronchial edema, produce bronchial wall thickening and indistinctness of the vascular margins. At the level of the secondary pulmonary lobule, disease in the axial interstitium produces tiny dots or Y-shaped opacities – the so-called centrilobular opacities. The peripheral interstitial tissue or shell of the lung is composed of the visceral pleura and its invaginations into the pulmonary fissures and extensions into the lung, which divide the lungs into lobes, segments and subsegments. Portions of the peripheral interstitium form the interlobular septa, which generally delineate the secondary pulmonary lobules. The pulmonary veins and lymphatics travel in the interlobular septa thickening of which are the source of the well-known Kerley B and A lines. Some lymphatics also travel in the bronchovascular bundles.

The secondary pulmonary lobule was described in detail by Heitzman et al. [16] who years ago suggested that recognition of this structure would aid in categorizing and understanding pulmonary disease. The secondary pulmonary lobule is a polyhedral structure about 1.5 to 2.0 cm in size. These lobules are much better formed in the periphery of the lung especially in the lower lobe than elsewhere. The structure of a lobule repeats the core and shell structure of the lung itself. The shell is formed by the interlobular septa, the core is composed of a peripheral pulmonary arterial branch and its accompanying terminal bronchial, which gives rise to an average of 5 to 8 pulmonary acini. The acinus is composed of strictly gas exchanging airways, the respiratory bronchioles, alveolar ducts and sacs. These structures in turn are closely related to a mesh-like web of capillaries and supported by the septal interstitium. Disease in this location is manifest on HRCT as ground-glass opacities, which because of the microscopic proximity of air space and interstitial tissues often makes the distinction between air space and interstitial diseases impossible [17].

Analysis of CT Findings of Pulmonary Disease

Most authors of HRCT papers agree that recognition of the secondary pulmonary lobule is useful in describing the type of disease which may then be classified as centrilobular, perilobular or panlobular [18-22]. If there is centrilobular disease, multiple ill-defined dots or Y-shaped structures are seen (centrilobular opacities). Their position in the center of the lobule is inferred by their size and shape. If interlobular septal thickening or venous prominence is present, many interlobular septa are seen and a linear or polygonal pattern of perilobular disease is present. Panlobular involvement is diagnosed if the entire secondary lobule is abnormal. In this case, a pattern of sharply delineated regions of attenuation differing from neighbouring lobules is readily recognized.

Air Space and Interstitial Disease

Air Space Disease

In addition to classifying CT findings by reference to the secondary pulmonary lobule, some authors also advocate the more traditional divisions of air space and interstitial disease. The findings of air space disease are those familiar from plain radiography. Air space (acinar) nodules, ground-glass opacities, consolidation, and air bronchograms are seen. Ground-glass opacities are defined as a localized increase in lung attenuation which still allows visualization of vascular structures coursing through the affected region [23]. These opacities may indicate early air space disease, but because of the intimate relationship between the air spaces and the septal interstitial tissues, they can also be a sign of early interstitial disease and may indicate alveolitis. Ground-glass opacities may reflect early and often treatable disease. They are panlobular in distribution.

Interstitial Disease

The classical CT signs of interstitial disease are related to the three types of pulmonary interstitium. Disease in the axial interstitium results in the presence of peribronchial vascular bundle thickening and centrilobular opacities. Disease in the peripheral interstitium produces Kerley lines, the "interface" sign, visceral pleural thickening and eventually honeycombing. Abnormality of the septal interstitium is manifest on HRCT by ground-glass opacities. Signs of chronic irreversible interstitial disease include thick parenchymal bands, honeycombing, larger lung cysts and advanced bronchiectasis.

CT Findings in Specific Pediatric Diseases

Importance of the Chest Radiograph and History

Despite the exquisite anatomy displayed by CT, the chest radiograph and history remain the most important factors in radiologic evaluation of pediatric pulmonary disease and the CT examination must always be inter-

preted in conjunction with this information. Currently it is unclear when CT will prove to be clinically useful for many diseases. In this section, I will attempt to summarize the CT findings in pediatric diseases that we or others have studied without attempting to defend or analyse the utility of CT in the specified conditions. Controlled studies and much more experience will be required before any conclusions can be reached regarding CT's ultimate role. Preliminary experience strongly suggests that CT is useful in the following situations: (1) evaluation of an apparently normal chest X-ray in a patient who has significant clinical symptoms; (2) clarification of an abnormal appearing but nonspecific chest X-ray; (3) evaluation of bronchiectasis; (4) evaluation of suspected metastatic disease; and (5) as a guide to biopsy and for evaluation of therapy. It is also evident that CT is able to diagnose small airways disease and shows potential for studying the effects of infection on the growing lung. It may have some utility in the staging of cystic fibrosis and the determination of the extent of bronchopulmonary dysplasia.

Diseases Associated with Multiple Pulmonary Nodules

Included in this grouping would be metastatic disease, pulmonary spread of laryngeal papillomatosis, fungal infection, tuberculosis, septic emboli, vasculitis and bronchiolitis obliterans with organizing pneumonia (BOOP). In children, pulmonary metastatic disease is usually secondary to a well-known primary disease and usually presents no difficulty in differential diagnosis. The nodules are frequently identified at the end of vessels and usually do not cavitate. Septic pulmonary emboli tend to be peripheral in nature and often may show cavitation. The source of infection is not infrequently hidden but most often is due to osteomyelitis or septic thrombophlebitis [24, 25]. As with metastatic disease, the primary condition is usually well-established in laryngeal papillomatosis. The papillomatous lesions seed down the large airways and into the periphery of the lung where they very frequently show cavitation.

Bronchiolitis obliterans with organizing pneumonia (BOOP) is an interesting entity, probably underdiagnosed in pediatrics [26-28]. It presents with patchy peripheral nodules which are often bilateral. The CT appearance is due to the visualization of the organizing pneumonia and not the areas of bronchiolitis obliterans. The condition may follow infection and is often associated with malignancy or altered immune status. It has been associated with bleomycin therapy [29, 30].

Larger Conglomerate Nodules and Ill-defined Pulmonary Masses

When visualized, large nodules and ill-defined pulmonary masses, suggest vasculitis. They may be associated with other findings of vasculitis including ground-glass opacities along the margins of the consolidated area producing a so-called "fried-egg" appearance [31]. This pattern is seen with invasive aspergillosis, malignancy, lymphomatoid granulomatosis and Wegener's granulomatosis. Invasive aspergillosis is usually associated with immune suppressive therapy for malignancy. Lymphomatoid granulomatosis is probably a form of T-cell lymphoma that affects the lung, skin and central nervous system while sparing the peripheral lymph nodes. It produces a mononuclear cell infiltrate associated with parenchymal necrosis and a perivascular infiltrate [32]. Wegener's granulomatosis usually presents in teenage children and is associated with glomerulonephritis and respiratory tract lesions including cavitating pulmonary masses or nodules [13, 33]. Diagnosis is established by detecting the presence of antineutrophil cytoplasmic antibodies [34]. The condition is sometimes responsive to Cytoxan and steroids. Langerhan's cell histiocytosis presents with small ill-defined nodules and thick- or thin-walled cysts [35-37]. The cysts may be peripheral and have an upper lobe predominance in adults although this pattern seems less common in childhood. The nodules are due to peribronchiocellular infiltrates. Thick-walled cysts may develop from cavitation of nodules. Thin-walled cysts may become confluent with the development of fibrosis and a honeycomb appearance in the lungs; their aetiology is controversial but may be due to an obstructive, check-valve phenomenon. The reticular findings often seen on plain chest radiography are shown on chest CT to be due to a combination of cysts and nodules. At least in some cases, the cysts in children appear to resolve without any significant pulmonary sequelae.

Ground-glass Opacities

As noted above, GGO can be due to either interstitial or air space disease and represent involvement of the septal portion of the pulmonary interstitium or air-space disease. A ground-glass appearance may be present in a segment of normal lung if an adjacent segment is hyperinflated. True GGO are due to alveolitis and diffuse alveolar damage, some forms of atypical pneumonia, especially pneumocystis carina and leukemic infiltrates. Early pulmonary oedema and haemorrhage also produce GGO. Pulmonary alveolar proteinosis is an uncommon pediatric disease that is classically associated with GGO and interlobular septal thickening.

Pulmonary alveolar proteinosis appears to consist of two distinct types. The later onset type may occur in later childhood or adults. It is not clear if this is the same disease as the congenital variant but it seems unlikely. Occasionally it responds to bronchoalveolar lavage. The infantile type of pulmonary alveolar proteinosis, also called congenital pulmonary alveolar proteinosis, has its onset at birth and may be an autosomal recessive condi-

tion. It causes respiratory failure which is progressive and nearly always fatal. Radiologically, it resembles respiratory distress syndrome and it may be due to a congenital deficiency of the presence of surfactant B [38].

In the adult type, the chest radiograph shows bilateral symmetric air space disease that looks like severe pulmonary oedema although the heart is normal. Some nodularity may be present at the margins. Interstitial markings are not prominent on the chest radiograph. HRCT shows diffuse GGO which have a sharp geometric pattern. Also associated with this is a very prominent pattern of smooth interlobular septal thickening. Septal thickening is probably due to oedema as biopsy in early cases shows no evidence of interstitial fibrosis.

Lymphangiectic Metastatic Disease

When the HRCT findings include thickening of the bronchovascular bundles, nodular septal thickening and discreet nodules and masses lymphangiectic metastatic disease is suspected. This pattern occurs in neuroblastoma, metastatic sarcoma and lymphoma, especially large cell lymphoma. Large cell lymphoma is frequently associated with a rapid onset of findings, a mediastinal mass, hilar nodes, pleural effusion and the above-described lymphangiectic pattern.

Small Airways Disease

Small airways are defined as the terminal bronchioles, respiratory bronchioles and alveolar ducts. While these structures are invisible on high resolution CT, disease of them is suggested by the following findings: (1) air-trapping that may be focal and only seen on expiratory CT images [39, 40] or; (2) diffuse and manifest by increased lung volumes suggested by the presence of prominent anterior and posterior junction lines. Focal pulmonary hyperlucency may be due to the air-trapping itself or to secondary affects of hypoxic vasoconstriction and shunting. Areas of focal pulmonary hyperlucency can be adjacent to areas of apparent GGO (mosaic perfusion pattern) [41, 42], but in this instance the regions of GGO are actually the normal lung that is of increased attenuation due to loss of volume by compression from adjacent hyperinflated lung and accentuated by shunting of blood from the hyperinflated lung.

Centrilobular Disease

Centrilobular disease is due to involvement of the terminal bronchioles, and is therefore another indicator of small airway disease [43]. Involvement of the terminal bronchioles produces a CT pattern of dots and Ys or the so-called "tree–in-bud"appearance [44]. Common causes of centrilobular opacities in children include cystic fibrosis, asthma particularly when complicated by infection, and infection of the small airways including mycoplasma pneumonia, bronchopneumonia, viral pneumonia and tuberculosis [45-47]. Uncommon conditions producing centrilobular opacities include BOOP, hypersensitivity pneumonia, early pulmonary oedema and occasionally malignancy.

Of these diseases, *cystic fibrosis* has been the most widely studied. It is a disease which begins in the airways and is manifest with findings of bronchial wall disease including centrilobular opacities, mucoid impaction, small airways disease with air-trapping and a mosaic perfusion or GGO pattern. Eventually, cystic bronchiectasis of a severe degree develops. The role of CT in evaluation of children with cystic fibrosis is as yet uncertain [48]. Clearly, CT can diagnose pulmonary involvement earlier than chest X-ray and may be helpful in children who are too young to participate in pulmonary function tests. It can stage disease more accurately than chest X-ray and it has been shown that there is good correlation with pulmonary function [49, 50]. CT may also be useful to follow effectiveness of therapy particularly in children on experimental protocols.

Bronchial Asthma. Bronchial asthma is much more common than cystic fibrosis but it is not usually studied with CT [51]. There has been no prospective study done of children with asthma although we have scanned many asthmatic children for a variety of reasons. Common findings include pulmonary hyperinflation, bronchial wall thickening and centrilobular opacities especially when complicated by infection. Bronchiectasis is uncommon. Marked mosaic perfusion patterns are occasionally visualized especially in younger children who have wheezing associated with bronchiolitis.

Obliterative Bronchiolitis. Obliterative bronchiolitis is a condition whose prevalence is unknown. Clinically, these affected children present with what is often thought to be reactive airways disease and recurrent infection. Severe cases may show unilateral hyperlucent lung (Swyer-James syndrome) on conventional chest radiography but CT usually shows multifocal disease [52, 53]. Obliterative bronchiolitis has multiple aetiologies but most commonly is due to sequela of a previous viral infection [54]. It is also commonly associated with post-transplant conditions as a manifestation of graft versus host disease [55, 56]. As opposed to bronchiolitis obliterans with organizing pneumonia, lung biopsy of obliterative bronchiolitis reveals that the terminal bronchioles are irreversibly narrowed by intramural fibrosis [57]. CT in this condition usually shows multifocal air-trapping with regions that are sharply marginated especially on expiration. The blood vessels are small, there may be mild associated bronchiectasis and centrilobular opacities [58]. At present, CT cannot differentiate findings of obliterative bronchiolitis from those due to reactive airways disease. An interval examination with little change favours obliterative bronchiolitis as does the presence of bronchiectasis. The exact relationship of obliterative bronchiolitis to bronchiectasis also remains obscure [59]. It is not known whether obliterative bronchiolitis precedes and causes bronchiectasis or if bronchiectasis may cause obliterative bronchiolitis. Certainly, multiple pathologic studies have shown that bronchiectasis is associated with obliterative bronchiolitis. Also unknown is how often obliterative bronchiolitis may occur following infection especially in the growing lung [54]. We have seen several instances of apparent obliterative bronchiolitis following infection and suspect that it may be significantly more common than is currently appreciated.

Interstitial disease that is chronic and irreversible is fortunately relatively uncommon in pediatrics [60, 61]. CT in affected patients reveals the presence of parenchymal bands, honeycombing, larger lung cysts and advanced bronchiectasis although the patterns differ [62]. This combination of findings occurs in children with advanced cystic fibrosis, late stages of adult respiratory distress syndrome, bronchopulmonary dysplasia and in some cases of Langerhan's cell histiocytosis, collagen vascular disease, neurocutaneous syndromes and idiopathic interstitial pulmonary fibrosis. The findings of bronchopulmonary dysplasia on CT include anterior fibrosis, increased lung volumes, lower lobe hyperinflation and areas of focal air-trapping, which may be due to bronchiolitis obliterans and emphysema, either primary or compensatory [63].

In conclusion, high resolution CT is very helpful in clarifying confusing radiographic findings and providing a more precise evaluation of disease extent. The separation of interstitial from air space disease is not always possible but a dominant CT pattern may often successfully allow categorization of disease. At the least, CT narrows the differential diagnosis, increases diagnostic confidence and can guide biopsy in cases where this is indicated [64].

References

1. Webb WR, Stein MG, Finkbeiner WE, et al. (1988) Normal and diseased isolated lungs: high-resolution CT. Radiology 166: 81
2. Bessis L, Callard P, Gotheil C, Biaggi A, Grenier P (1992) High-resolution CT of parenchymal lung disease: precise correlation with histologic findings. Radiographics 12: 45-58
3. Kuhn JP (1993) High-resolution computed tomography of pediatric pulmonary parenchymal disorders. Radiol Clin North Am 31: 533-551
4. Moon WK, Kim WS, Kim IO, Im JG, Yeon KM, Han MC (1996) Diffuse pulmonary disease in children: high-resolution CT findings. AJR 167: 1405-1408
5. Seely JM, Effmann EL, Muller NL (1997) High-resolution CT of pediatric lung disease: imaging findings. AJR 168: 1269-1275
6. Kuhn JP, Slovis TL, Silverman FN, Kuhns LR (1993) The neck and respiratory system. In: Silverman FN, Kuhn JP (eds) Caffey's pediatric X-ray diagnosis. Mosby, St. Louis, pp 345-697

7. Webb WR, Muller NL, Naidich DP (1996) High-resolution CT of the lung, 2nd ed. Lippincott-Raven, New York, pp 4-13

8. Mayo JR, Webb WR, Gould R, et al. (1987) High-resolution CT of the lungs: an optimal approach. Radiology 163: 507

9. Murata K, Khan A, Rojas KA, et al. (1988) Optimization of computed tomography technique to demonstrate the fine structure of the lung. Invest Radiol 23: 170

10. Naidich DP, Marshal CH, Gribbin C, et al. (1990) Low-dose CT of the lungs: preliminary observations. Radiology 175: 729

11. Ambrosino MM, Genieser NB, Roche KJ, Kaul A, Lawrence RM (1994) Feasibility of high-resolution, low-dose chest CT in evaluating the pediatric chest. Pediatr Radiol 24: 6-10

12. Naidich DP, Muller NL, Zerhouni EA, Webb WR, Krinsky GA, Siegelman SS, McGuinness G (1999) Computed tomography and magnetic resonance of the thorax. Lippincott-Raven, Philadelphia, pp 1-16

13. Kuhlman JE, Hruban RH, Fishman EK (1991) Wegener granulomatosis: CT features of parenchymal lung disease. J Comput Assist Tomogr 15: 948-952

14. Weibel ER, Bachofen H (1991) The fiber scaffold of lung parenchyma. In: Crystal RG, West JB (eds) The lung, Vol. 1. Raven Press, New York, pp 787-794

15. Weibel ER, Crystal RG (1991) Structural organization of the pulmonary interstitium. In: Crystal RG, West JB (eds) The lung, Vol. 1. Raven Press, New York, pp 369-380

16. Heitzman ER, Markarian B, Berger I, et al. (1969) The secondary pulmonary lobule: a practical concept for interpretation of chest radiographs. Radiology 93: 507-519

17. Bergin C, Roggli V, Coblentz C, et al. (1988) The secondary pulmonary lobule: normal and abnormal CT appearances. AJR 151: 21

18. Galvin JR, Mori M, Stanford W (1992) High-resolution computed tomography and diffuse lung disease. Curr Probl Diag Radiol 21: 31-74

19. Lynch DA, Brasch RC, Hardy KA, et al. (1990) Pediatric pulmonary disease: assessment with high-resolution ultrafast CT. Radiology 176: 243

20. Naidich DP, Zerhouni EA, Hutchins GM, et al. (1985) Computed tomography of the pulmonary parenchyma: Part 2. Interstitial disease. J Thorac Imaging 1: 54

21. Naidich DP, Zerhouni EA, Hutchins GM, et al. (1985) Computed tomography of the pulmonary parenchyma: Part 1. Distal air-space disease. J Thorac Imaging 1: 39

22. Kuhn JP (1991) Pediatric thorax In: Naidich DP, Zerhouni EA, Siegelman S (eds) Computed tomography and magnetic resonance of the thorax, 2nd ed. Raven Press, New York, pp 503-555

23. Collins J, Stern EJ (1997) Ground-glass opacity at CT: the ABCs. AJR 169: 355-367

24. De Sena S, Rosenfeld DL, Santos S, Keller I (1996) Jugular thrombophlebitis complicating bacterial pharyngitis (Lemierre's syndrome). Pediatr Radiol 26: 141-144

25. Gudinchet F, Maeder P, Neveceral P, Schnyder P (1997) Lemierre's syndrome in children. High-resolution CT and color Doppler sonography patterns. Chest 112: 271-273

26. Helton KJ, Kuhn JP, Fletcher BD, et al. (1992) Bronchiolitis obliterans: organizing pneumonia (BOOP) in children with malignant disease. Pediatr Radiol 22: 270-274

27. Akira M, Yamamoto S, Sakatani M (1998) Bronchiolitis obliterans organizing pneumonia manifesting as multiple large nodules or masses. AJR 170: 291-295

28. Inoue T, Toyoshima K, Kikui M (1996) Idiopathic bronchiolitis obliterans organizing pneumonia (idiopathic BOOP) in childhood. Pediatr Pulmonol 22: 67-72

29. Arush MWB, Roguin A, Zamir E, El-Hassid R, Pries D, Gaitini D, Dale A, Postovsky S (1997) Bleomycin and cyclophosphamide toxicity simulating metastatic nodules to the lungs in childhood cancer. Pediatr Hematol Oncol 14: 381-386

30. D'Alessandro MP, Kozakewich HPW, Cooke KR, Taylor GA (1996) Radiologic-pathologic conference of children's hospital Boston: new pulmonary nodules in a child undergoing treatment for a solid malignancy. Pediatr Radiol 26: 19-21

31. Logan PM, Primack SL, Miller RR, Muller NL (1994) Invasive aspergilliosis of the airways: radiographic, CT, and pathologic findings. Radiology 193: 383-388

32. Pearson ADJ, Kirpalani H, Ashcroft T, Bain H, Craft AW (1983) Lymphomatoid granulomatosis in a 10 year old boy. BMJ 286: 1313-1314

33. Wadsworth DT, Siegel MJ, Day DL (1994) Wegener's granulomatosis in children: chest radiographic manifestations. AJR 163: 901-905

34. Baldree LA, Gaber LW, McKay CP (1991) Anti-neutrophil cytoplasmic autoantibodies in a child with pauciimmune necrotizing and crescentic glomerulonephritis. Pediatr Nephrol 5: 296-299

35. Brauner MW, Grenier P, Tijani K, Battesti JP, Valeyre D (1997) Pulmonary Langerhans cell histiocystosis: evolution of lesions on CT scans. Radiology 204: 497-502

36. Ha SY, Helms P, Fletcher M, Broadbent V, Pritchard J (1992) Lung involvement in Langerhans cell histiocytosis: prevalence, clinical features, and outcome. Pediatrics 89: 466-469

37. Kulwiec EL, Lynch DA, Aguayo SM, Schwarz MI, King TE Jr (1992) Imaging of pulmonary histiocytosis X. Radiographics 12: 515-526

38. Nogee LM, deMello DE, Dehner LP, Colten HR (1993) Brief report: deficiency of pulmonary surfactant protein B in congenital alveolar proteinosis. N Engl J Med 328: 406-410

39. Hansell DM, Rubens MB, Padley SP, Wells AU (1997) Obliterative bronchiolitis: individual CT signs of small airways disease and functional correlation. Radiology 203: 721-726

40. Desai SR, Hansell DM (1997) Small airways disease: expiratory computed tomography comes of age. Clin Radiol 52: 332-337

41. Stern EJ, Muller NL, Swensen SJ, Hartman TE (1995) CT mosaic pattern of lung attenuation: etiologies and terminology. J Thorac Imaging 10: 294-297

42. Stern EJ, Swensen SJ, Hartman TE, Frank MS (1995) CT mosaic pattern of lung attenuation: distinguishing different cases. AJR 165: 813-816

43. Gruden JF, Webb WR, Warnock M (1994) Centrilobular opacities in the lung on high-resolution CT: diagnostic considerations and pathologic correlation. AJR 162: 569-574

44. Aquino SL, Gamsu G, Webb WR, Kee ST (1996) Tree-in-bud pattern: frequency and significance on thin section CT. J Comput Assist Tomogr 20: 594-599

45. Tanaka N, Matsumoto T, Kuramitsu T, Nakaki H, Ito K, Uchisako H, Miura G, Matsunaga N, Yamakawa K (1996) High resolution CT findings in community-acquired pneumonia. J Comput Assist Tomogr 20: 600-608

46. Jamieson DH, Cremin BJ (1993) High resolution CT of the lungs in acute disseminated tuberculosis and a pediatric radiology perspective of the term "miliary". Pediatr Radiol 23: 380-383

47. Kim WS, Moon WK, Kim IO, Lee HJ, Im JG, Yeon KM, Han MC (1997) Pulmonary tuberculosis in children: evaluation with CT. AJR 168: 1005-1009

48. Santamaria F, Grillo G, Guidi G, Rotondo A, Raia V, de Ritis G, Sarnelli P, Caterino M, Greco L (1998) Cystic fibrosis: when should high-resolution computed tomography of the chest be obtained? Pediatrics 101: 908-913

49. Nathanson I, Conboy K, Murphy S, Kuhn J (1991) Ultrafast computerized tomography of the chest in cystic fibrosis. Pediatr Pulmonol 11: 81

50. Bhalla M, Turcios N, Aponte V, et al. (1991) Cystic fibrosis: scoring system with thin-section CT. Radiology 179: 783
51. Lynch DA, Newell JD, Tschomper BA, Cink TM, Newman LS, Bethel R (1993) Uncomplicated asthma in adults: comparison of CT appearance of the lungs in asthmatic and healthy subjects. Radiology 188: 829-833
52. Hansell DAM, Rubens MB, Padley SPG, Wells AU (1997) Obliterative bronchiolitis: individual CT signs of small airways disease and functional correlation. Radiology 203: 721-726
53. Marti-Bonmati L, Perales FR, Catala F, et al. (1989) CT findings in Swyer-James syndrome. Radiology 172: 477
54. Chang AB, Masel JP, Masters B (1998) Post-infectious bronchiolitis obliterans: clinical, radiological and pulmonary function sequelae. Pediatr Radiol 28: 23-29
55. Sargent MA, Cairns RA, Murdoch MJ, Nadel HR, Wensley D, Schultz KR (1995) Obstructive lung disease in children after allogeneic bone marrow transplantation: evaluation with high-resolution CT. AJR 164: 693-696
56. Worthy SA, Flint JD, Muller NL (1997) Pulmonary complications after bone marrow transplantation: high-resolution CT and pathologic findings. Radiographics 17: 1359-1371
57. Garg K, Lynch DA, Newell JD, King TE Jr (1994) Prolifer-
ative and constrictive bronchiolitis: classification and radiologic features. AJR 162: 803-808
58. Stern EJ, Frank MS (1994) Small-airway diseases of the lungs: findings at expiratory CT. AJR 163: 37-41
59. Hansell DM, Wells AU, Rubens MB, Cole PJ (1994) Bronchiectasis: functional significance of areas of decreased attenuation at expiratory CT. Radiology 193: 369-374
60. Katzenstein ALA, Gordon LP, Oliphant M, Swender PT (1995) Chronic pneumonitis of infancy. A unique form of interstitial lung disease occurring in early childhood. Am J Surg Pathol 19: 439-447
61. Fan LL (1994) Evaluation and therapy of chronic interstitial pneumonitis in children. Curr Opin Pediatr 6: 248-254
62. Muller NL, Coiby TV (1997) Idiopathic interstitial pneumonias: high-resolution CT and histologic findings. Radiographics 17: 1016-1022
63. Oppenheim C, Mamou-Mani T, Sayegh N, de Blic J, Scheinmann P, Lallemand D (1994) Bronchopulmonary dysplasia: value of CT in identifying pulmonary sequelae. AJR 163: 169-172
64. Spencer DA, Alton HM, Raafat F, Weller PH (1996) Combined percutaneous lung biopsy and high-resolution computed tomography in the diagnosis and management of lung disease in children. Pediatr Pulmonol 22: 111-116

SESSION II

Modern Imaging in the Follow-up of Brain Tumor Therapy

S. Neuenschwander

Department of Radiology and Nuclear Medicine, Institut Curie, Paris, France

Introduction

During the last decade, the management of brain tumor has changed considerably: modern surgical techniques, including computer-assisted resection, permit a greater degree of resection in a larger number of patients, reducing neurological damage [1, 2]. New radiation therapy techniques attempt to escalate the dose of radiation without increasing the risk of radiation-induced toxicity. These techniques include hyperfractionation, three-dimensional conformal treatment planning, interstitial brachytherapy, radiosurgery, fractionated stereotaxic radiotherapy, and proton beam therapy. All these sophisticated therapeutic possibilities imply a precise delineation of the target, with pretreatment planning optimally using 3D, image fusion and simulation.

On the other hand, high-dose small-field radiation therapy increases the likelihood of radiation necrosis, creating diagnostic difficulties on follow-up imaging studies. Concurrently, chemotherapy regimens are being increasingly used in surgically nonaccessible tumors or after surgery, especially in children less than 3 or 5 years of age, in order to delay or even avoid radiotherapy. New drugs that may stabilize the blood brain barrier or modulators of tumor neovascularity are under investigation. All these protocols require methods to monitor tumor activity. Facing these challenges, what can we provide?

Modalities

Classical. Computed tomography (CT) and magnetic resonance imaging (MRI) scans are routinely used in the follow-up of brain tumors during and after treatment. Although MRI is able to provide fine anatomical detail, allowing good targeting of the lesion, its lack of specificity, for example in differentiating tumor recurrence from post-therapeutic gliosis [3], compel to finding new methods.

Functional. "Physiological" imaging may have the potential to differentiate neoplastic from nonneoplastic brain tissue:

- *Single-photon emission computed tomography (SPECT)* with Thallium-201 (^{201}Tl) relies on the uptake and/or metabolism of a radioactive tracer to identify high grade tumor components. Thallium is an analog of potassium, possessing a higher affinity for the Na and K-activated adenosine triphosphatase pump and a slower wash-out from cells than potassium. It collects avidly into viable dividing cells. High grade gliomas demonstrate intense uptake, although low grade gliomas show only a marginal increase of the radiopharmaceutical uptake [4]. ^{201}Tl uptake and retention has been used to distinguish glioma recurrence from radiation necrosis. If false negative results due to the small size, the type or the low grade of the lesion may occur [5], false positive results have also been reported in radiation necrosis [6, 7].

- *Positron emission tomography (PET)* provides functional information about the brain, either hemodynamic data (blood flow, blood volume) or metabolic (glucose, oxygen use, protein synthesis). Administrated compounds are labeled with positron emitters (i.e., ^{18}F, ^{11}C). The physical principle is the detection of two photons produced after the anihilation of an emitted positron with an electron. Collected data produced the 20-40 slices of tomographic images simultaneously. Intrinsic detection resolution is 4-6 mm.

- *[^{18}F] 2-deoxy-2 fluoro D glucose (FDG) PET:* The theoretical basis is that tumor cells have increased glucose metabolism (high rate of aerobic glycolysis), whereas irradiated cells have decreased glucose utilization. After encouraging preliminary studies, recent papers report low specificity (22-56%) in its ability to differentiate recurrent tumor from radiation necrosis [8, 9]. A better indication might be tumor monitoring under chemotherapy [10].

- *Methionine, tyrosine and choline labeled PET* scanning are newer technologies that are based on amino acid membrane transport, protein synthesis and phospholipid uptake. They might have interest for low grade, nonenhancing brain gliomas with low glucose consumption, and therefore permit residual tumor detection [11]. An increased tracer uptake has been demonstrated in some childhood tumors, like medulloblastoma, ependymoma and astrocytoma [12]. Although potentially more accurate than FDG PET, these methods are costly and still of limited availability.

Radionuclide-based techniques generally have poorer spatial resolution than the MRI-based techniques. The synergistic use of different modalities, optimally with image fusion, allow each method to be used to its full advantage. Image fusion leads to increased precision in anatomico-functional correlation, and becomes a valuable tool when planning surgery or radiation therapy [13, 14], or in identifying relapse after treatment.

- *Perfusion-weighted MR* techniques are sensitive to microscopic anounts of blood flow. In dynamic gadolinium enhanced relative cerebral blood volume (rCBV) imaging, the T2 MRI signal drop in a brain region is caused by spin dephasing from susceptibility effects during a rapid passage of the paramagnetic contrast medium through the capillary bed. Perfusion imaging maps are ideally performed using echo planar imaging, but may be also obtained with conventional MR scanners. Perfusion imaging provides a map of tumor perfusion: highly vascular tumors have high rCBV values, whereas others, like medulloblastoma, demonstrate low rCBV [15]. Some glial tumors that do not enhance with gadolinium may still have anaplastic features: this is the reason why high CBV foci may be found in nonenhancing tumors. Moreover, in rapidly growing tumors or postradiation therapy lesions, leaky regions of brain blood barrier rupture alter the rCBV values and this effect has to be compensated before mapping. In these situations, other techniques, such as T1-based absolute flow methods are valuable. Perfusion MR imaging might monitor the local microcirculation and consequently the effects of new treatment restricting tumor angiogenesis. Pilot studies in adult gliomas have suggested that perfusion MR may be as effective as radionuclide-based techniques in sensitivity and specificity when assessing brain tumor response to therapy [15], and even superior, especially for lesions smaller than 1.5 cm [16]. Their effectiveness in management of pediatric brain tumors remains to be proven.
- *Proton magnetic resonance spectroscopy (MRS)* may be added to routine MRI to provide noninvasive brain biochemistry, measuring the major brain neurotransmitters and metabolites. Several conditions are essential for obtaining interpretable biochemical data: avoidance of motion artifacts or metal containing orthodontic braces, optimal shimming (magnetic field homogeneity) and water suppression adjustment. To quantify spectral data, the most common method uses metabolite ratios, although a water-referencing approach may prove to be more sensitive and specific

[17]. High grade brain tumors tend to have increased levels of choline. Thus, it is theoretically possible to differentiate a recurrence (high level of choline with easily visible creatine metabolites) and radiation necrosis (marked depression of the intracellular metabolite peaks from choline, creatine and N acetyl compounds) [18]. Recently, the use of short-echo-time proton MRS has allowed macromolecules and lipids to be observed: lipids have also been recognized as potential indicators of malignancy. High lactate levels can be found in malignant and benign tumors: a recent report on pediatric pilocytic astrocytomas indicates the detection of a lactate signal in 8 of 8 patients [19]. However, most of the MRS pediatric literature is based on tumor characterization and there is little information about its use for the follow up.

Problems

Postsurgical Modification/Residual Tumor

For many brain tumors, incomplete resection directly affects the therapeutic management. Thus, the main challenge of postoperative imaging is to assess the existence of residual tumor. As an early postoperative MRI is difficult to obtain in some countries for logistic reasons, the reference examination is still often a CT scanner: it has to be performed within 48 h of surgery, with pre- and postcontrast medium images. This technique allows hemorrhage to be differentiated from contrast enhancement. In the first hours following surgery, contrast medium leakage due to extravasation into the tumor resection cavity can be detected [20]. On early CT scans, within 48 h of surgery, contrast enhancement at the edge of the operative site is indicative of residual tumor [21, 22]. Contrast enhancement resulting from surgical trauma appears later and can persist for several months.

Early postoperative MRI demonstrates slightly different patterns, as shown by Forsyth et al. [23] in a series of adult gliomas: nonneoplastic linear contrast enhancement at the edge of the surgical cavity could be detected, although faint, as early as day 1 and was maximal between days 5 to 14 after surgery; tumor enhancement was optimally visualized on postoperative days 3 to 5; methemoglobin was the most unpredictable parameter, mainly present between days 7 and 21, but in some cases interfering with early residual tumor assessment. Accelerated methemoglobin formation might be in relation with hydrogen peroxide used in neurosurgery [24]. Elster and DiPersio, in a study of 50 postoperative MRI scans, confirmed that marginal enhancement at the operative site is visualized earlier with MRI than with CT scan and can persist up to 1 year [25]; postsurgical nonneoplastic meningeal enhancement may also persist for several years. Although everyone agrees that MRI is more sensitive than CT and with the principle of early assessment, the optimal date recommended for MRI varies between days 1 to 3, and 3 to 5, depending on the authors [25, 26].

Monitoring Tumoral Activity

In clinical practice, the follow-up of nonresectable or residual tumor is based on clinical status and on *comparative measurements* of the lesion on successive contrast enhanced MRI. Several pitfalls have to be avoided: corticosteroid therapy, given for symptoms of intracranial hypertension, may induce a false appreciation of tumor volume variation, as shown by Watling et al. [27]. The contrast enhancement and the hypersignal on T2-weighted images may be reduced by up to 25% within the first 2 weeks of the treatment. Conversely, edema or inflammatory process induced by radiation treatment may increase the tumor size. On the other hand, low-grade tumors, such as hypothalamic/ chiasmatic astrocytomas, may on several successive exams show such subtle changes that they would be noticeable only if the pretreatment exams were considered for comparison.

From successive MRI, attempts have been made to elaborate mathematical models of brain tumor growth [28, 29]. Their theoretical advantage could be to provide a better idea of the tumor proliferation and infiltration. Although the most used in practice, the variation in tumor size is not a sufficient criteria to appreciate tumor activity.

The appearance or the increase of a *contrast enhanced lesion* is always considered an alarm sign: however, posttreatment lesions may enhance, while certain recurrences do not enhance, such as intraventricular relapse of medulloblastoma [30], or recurrent ependymomas.

In this context can *functional imaging* play a role? Recently, Molenkamp et al. [31] stressed the value of iodine 123-methylthyrosine SPECT in the follow-up of low grade glioma of childhood. Holthoff et al. [10] reported a pilot study of serial PET studies under chemotherapy of seven children with medulloblastoma/primitive neuroectodermal tumor (PNET). He found as a consistent observation that medulloblastomas have a specially high glucose metabolism rate. He also reported a good correlation between the decrease in tumor metabolism and the therapeutic effect: his data suggest that FDG-PET might play a specific role in evaluating early response to treatment.

Postradiotherapeutic (and/or Chemotherapeutic) Images/Recurrence

High-dose small-field radiation therapy increases the likelihood of radiation necrosis. In 1996, Barkadjiev et al. reported MRI changes after stereotactic radiation therapy for childhood low grade astrocytomas [32]: 43% of the children developed increased size of the lesion, increased signal intensity or enhancement, cysts or cavitation and increase in edema on follow-up imaging. These changes generally appeared without clinical symptoms and were transient: most occurred between 9 and 12 months after stereotactic radiation and decreased or resolved by 15 to 21 months. Interstitial irradiation also produces local changes: Moringlane et al. reported in some patients the appearance after 4 weeks of a low attenuation spheric structure 6-8 mm in diameter with an enhanced ring, representing tissue necrosis at the site of the temporary radioactive implant [33].

Some protocols combine *radiotherapy and concomitant chemotherapy:* Van Tassel et al. [34] studied a series of adults treated for malignant gliomas with accelerated fractionation radiation therapy and carboplatin chemotherapy; he described a pattern of unusual enhancing lesions, more extensive than focal necrotic lesions after conventional radiotherapy, representing necrosis and reactive gliosis.

Pediatric series also demonstrate the difficulties in follow-up imaging of common brain tumors during or after treatment [3, 35]. The most critical situations are clinical and MRI deterioration occurring several months after fractionation radiotherapy, or clinical deterioration with stable MRI under chemotherapy for progressive disease. Under these circumstances, functional imaging must be contemplated: unfortunately, in clinical practice, its sensitivity and specificity are still suboptimal and the diagnosis is eventually assessed by surgery if possible or by the evolution of the tumor.

Delayed Abnormalities

Postradiation vasculopathy is a well-known late complication: cerebral ischemia or spontaneous cerebral hemorrhage occurring several years after treatment can easily be connected with radiation therapy by reviewing the radiation fields. However, the significance of some abnormalities observed in long-term survivors remains unclear: white matter changes are now easily seen with MRI, but their exact correlation with the modalities of the therapeutic regimen and their clinical correspondence are not yet well understood.

Is it worth it?

Since the middle of the 1990s, several papers have tried to evaluate the benefit of routine surveillance imaging for monitoring children after treatment of brain tumors. Is there a benefit to diagnosing an asymptomatic recurrence? Repetitive surveillance examinations certainly contribute to anxiety in the family and also the morbidity associated with the sedation of a young child. Imaging is also costly and in many institutions competes with other indications because of scarce imaging time on these machines.

In 1994, Torres et al. [36] started the controversy by reviewing the clinical records of 86 children with posterior fossa medulloblastoma, which were regularly followed between 1980 and 1991. He concluded that surveillance scanning with CT or MR is of little clinical value because a minority of recurrence (4 of 23) was detected on scanning only, and no patient with recurrence survived in his series. He recommended limiting the scanning to the detection of change in tumoral status after therapy, and thereafter to perform imaging only on clinical indications. He admitted, however, that his conclusion may change if a cure was developed for recurrent medulloblastoma.

In a similar group of patients, Mendel et al. [37] reported different results: in his series he assessed that asymptomatic patients with recurrence documented on serial imaging had prolonged survival compared with those who were symptomatic; thus, he concluded that early detection of local tumor recurrence may provide a critical therapeutic window for successful treatment with aggressive or novel therapies. Several commentaries about Torres' paper [38, 39] stressed the utility of an early detection of relapses considering new therapeutic possibilities: high dose myeloablative chemotherapies, and technological innovations in radiotherapy such as radiosurgery and brachytherapy.

Steinbock et al. [40] continued on this path, reporting a chart review of 159 children managed at a tertiary care hospital for various pediatric brain tumors: he concluded that during this study period, surveillance imaging was not valuable in identifying recurrence of cerebellar astrocytoma or supratentorial ganglioglioma, but was probably worthwhile in identifying recurrence of posterior fossa ependymoma, optic/hypothalamic astrocytoma and, possibly, medulloblastoma.

Our position at the Société Française d'Oncologie Pédiatrique (SFOP) is also that surveillance protocols could be made more effective by adapting them to each type of tumor, based on current data regarding the patterns of recurrence and the remaining therapeutic possibilities.

• In the case of low grade astrocytoma, recurrences often occur at the site of the primary tumor. For operable low grade astrocytomas, such as *cerebellar astrocytoma*, recurrence is unusual if the tumor has been completely resected; the discovery of a recurrence leads to a second surgical resection. As the favorable outcome is not influenced by an earlier diagnosis, the benefit of a surveillance seems to be poor. Sutton et al. [41] have proposed a model in which patients with possible or definite residual tumor after surgery undergo examinations at 12, 18, 30, 42 and 66 months. For them, this model would yield optimum predictive value for recurrence or progression with the fewest images.

In *optic/hypothalamic astrocytomas*, treatment is undertaken only in the case of visual deterioration or tumor growth at successive exams and surveillance is of major importance for the decision to treat, specially in the case of NF1. In the youngest patients, the new therapeutic approach is chemotherapy in order to postpone radiotherapy. Under these circumstances, surveillance is of major importance to evaluate the therapeutic efficacy and to change the treatment if necessary.

• In *high grade gliomas*, postoperative evaluation is crucial to assess tumor removal. In infants, imaging follow-up is worthwhile because a recurrence after chemotherapy leads to surgery and radiotherapy. In older children after radiotherapy, an imaging surveillance may be justified only if an inclusion in a phase II trial is contemplated.

• Recurrences of *ependymomas* mainly occur at the site of the primary tumor. The high risk period is from 18 months to more than 3.5 years after resection. Moreover, in Steinbock's study [40], fourth ventricular ependymoma stood out as the single tumor in which more than half of the recurrences were diagnosed by surveillance imaging. Infants not previously treated with radiotherapy must be carefully followed, because local recurrences may be efficaciously treated by a second operation followed by local radiotherapy. In children who have already received radiotherapy after surgery, chemotherapy has never demonstrated effectiveness, and surveillance would be justified only if new surgery is contemplated or if the patient were eligible for a novel therapeutic approach (phase I or II).

• The high risk period for *medulloblastoma/PNET* to recur is within 2.5 years after resection, especially the first 15 months, although late recurrence at more than 3 years is occasionally reported [42]. The frequency of asymptomatic recurrence is variable (from 17 to 62% in the literature), but the important factor is that they could be intracranial or intraspinal. Length of survival is primarily related to some specific patterns of relapse (time from diagnosis to recurrence, circumstances of relapse, extent of relapse) and to the response to salvage therapy [43]. At present, in this situation, the therapeutic possibilities depend on the risk factors at diagnosis and on the previous treatment: a standard risk medulloblastoma is defined as a primary tumor completely resected, without either suspected residual tumor at postoperative work-up or meningeal metastasis; high risk medulloblastoma is defined by residual primary tumor and/or meningeal metastasis.

– In infants with standard risk medulloblastoma who are treated only by surgery and chemotherapy, a second remission may be achieved using conventional and/or intensive chemotherapy, most often associated with posterior fossa radiation therapy.

– Infants with high risk medulloblastoma have a poor prognosis, and imaging follow up is justified to evaluate new therapeutic approaches.

- In older children with standard or high risk medulloblastoma, a monofocal relapse in the CNS may sometimes be actively treated with second line chemotherapy. Plurifocal relapse still carries a specially poor prognosis.

- The prognosis of *brain stem glioma* depends on whether the tumor is diffuse or focal: focal exophytic tumors have a relatively favorable prognosis regardless of the site of origin, while diffuse pontine tumors have the worst prognosis [44]. Over the last years, the main focus of research has been on the use of new techniques in radiation therapy, especially hyperfractionated radiotherapy. The effects of these treatments have to be evaluated. MR can also demonstrate tumor progression before clinical deterioration [45]. After treatment, surveillance imaging would be justified only in the case of trials.

Conclusion

Although the infant brain is more plastic in its response to surgical trauma, the effects of radiation therapy, and chemotherapy on vital developmental processes may have long-term consequences on motor, hormonal and intellectual functions. In infants as in older children, it is essential to provide the oncologists with accurate information on tumor status and treatment effects in order to change the therapy on time and, in favorable cases, reduce treatment related sequelae.

Acknowledgements. F. Doz, Pediatric Department, Institut Curie, Paris, France.

References

1. Nabavi A, Manthei G, Blomer U, Kumpf L, Klinge H, Mehdorn HM (1995) Neuronavigation. Computer-assisted surgery in neurosurgery. Radiology 35: 573-577
2. Zerah M, Druet H, Cinalli G, Brunelle F, Sainte Rose C (1998) Robotique et neurochirurgie 4: 137-144
3. Moghrabi A, Tien R, Fuchs H, Longee D, McLendon R, Friedman HS (1997) False positive images in the follow-up of patients with brain tumors. Med Pediatr Oncol 28: 127-131
4. Sjoholm H, Elmqvist D, Rehncrona S, Rosen I, Salford LG (1995) SPECT imaging of gliomas with Thallium-201 and Technetium 99m-HMPAO. Acta Neurol Scand 91: 66-70
5. Lorberboym M, Mandell LR, Mosesson RE, Germano I, et al. (1997) The role of thallium-201 uptake and retention in intracranial tumors after radiotherapy. J Nuclear Med 38: 223-226
6. Sonoda Y, Kumabe T, Takahashi T, Shirane R, Yoshimoto T (1998) Clinical usefulness of 11C-MET PET and 201T1 SPECT for differentiation of recurrent glioma from radiation necrosis. Neurol Med Chir 38: 342-348
7. Yoshii Y, Moritake T, Suzuki K, Fujita K, Nose T, Satou M (1996) Cerebral radiation necrosis with accumulation of thallium 201 on single-photon emission CT. AJNR 17: 1773-1776
8. Ricci PE, Karis JP, Heiserman JE, Fram EK, et al. (1998) Differentiating recurrent tumor from radiation necrosis: time for re-evaluation of positron emission tomography? AJNR 19: 407-413
9. Olivero WC, Dulebohn SC, Lister JR (1995) The use of PET in evaluating patients with primary brain tumours: is it useful? J Neurol Neurosurg Psychiatry 58: 250-252
10. Holthoff VA, Herholz K, Berthold F (1993) In vivo metabolism of childhood posterior fossa tumors and primitive neuroectodermal tumors before and after treatment. Cancer 72: 1394-1403
11. Herholz K, Hölzer T, Bauer B (1998) ^{11}C-methionine PET for differential diagnosis of low grade gliomas. Neurology 50: 1316-1322
12. O'Tuama LA, Phillips PC, Strauss LC, Carson BC, Uno Y, et al. (1990) Two-phase [11C]L-methionine PET in childhood brain tumors. Pediatr Neurol 6: 163-170
13. d'Asseler YM, Koole M, Lemahieu I, Achten E, et al. (1997) Recent and future evolutions in NeuroSPECT with particular emphasis on the synergistic use and fusion of imaging modalities. Acta Neurol Belg 97:154-162
14. Emri M, Esik O, Repa I, Marian T, Tron L (1997) Image fusion of different tomographic methods (PET/CT/MRI) effectively contribute to therapy planning. Orv Hetil 138: 2919-2924
15. Lev MH, Hochberg F (1998) Perfusion magnetic resonance imaging to assess brain tumor responses to new therapies. Cancer Control 5: 115-123
16. Siegal T, Rubinstein R, Tzuk-Shina T, Gomori JM (1997) Utility of relative cerebral blood volume mapping derived from perfusion magnetic resonance imaging in the routine follow up of brain tumors. J Neurosurg 86: 22-27
17. Moore GJ (1998) Proton magnetic resonance spectroscopy in pediatric neuroradiology. Pediatr Radiol 28: 805-814
18. Taylor JS, Langston JW, Reddick WE, et al. (1996) Clinical value of proton magnetic resonance spectroscopy for differentiating recurrent or residual brain tumor from delayed cerebral necrosis. Int J Radiat Oncol Biol Phys 36: 1251-1261
19. Hwang JH, Egnaczyk GF, Ballard E, et al. (1998) Proton MR spectroscopic characteristics of pediatric pilocytic astrocytomas. AJNR 19: 535-540
20. Spetzger U, Thron A, Gilsbach JM (1998) Immediate postoperative CT contrast enhancement following surgery of cerebral tumoral lesions. J Comput Assist Tomogr 22: 120-125
21. Nicoletti GF, Barone F, Passanisi M, Mancuso P, Albanese V (1994) Linear contrast enhancement at the operative site on early post-operative CT after removal of brain tumors. J Neurosurg Sci 38: 131-135
22. Bourne JP, Geyer R, Berger M, Griffin B, Milstein J (1992) The prognostic significance of postoperative residual contrast enhancement on CT scan in pediatric patients with medulloblastoma. J Neurooncol 14: 263-270
23. Forsyth PA, Petrov E, Mahallati H, Cairncross JG, Brasher P, et al. (1997) Prospective study of postoperative magnetic resonance imaging in patients with malignant gliomas. J Clin Oncol 15: 2076-2081
24. Meyding-Lamade U, Forsting M, Albert F, Kunze S, Sartor K (1993) Accelerated methaemoglobin formation: potential pitfall in early postoperative MRI. Neuroradiology 35: 178-180
25. Elster AD, DiPersio DA (1990) Cranial postoperative site: assessment with contrast-enhanced MR imaging. Radiology 174: 93-98
26. Albert FK, Forsting M, Sartor K, Adams HP, Kunze S (1994) Early postoperative magnetic resonance imaging after resection of malignant glioma: objective evaluation of residual tumor and its influence on regrowth and prognosis. Neurosurgery 34: 45-61
27. Watling CJ, Lee DH, Macdonald DR, et al. (1994) Corticos-

teroid-induced magnetic resonance imaging changes in patients with recurrent malignant glioma. J Clin Oncol 12: 1886-1889

28. Tracqui P, Cruywagen GC, Woodward DE, Bartoo GT, Murray JD, Alvord EC Jr (1995) A mathematical model of glioma growth: the effect of chemotherapy on spatio-temporal growth. Cell Prolif 28: 17-31

29. Tracqui P, Leitner F, Esteve (1995) Caractérisation dynamique de la croissance des tumeurs cérébrales à partir de séquences d'images obtenues par résonance magnétique nucléaire. Bull Cancer 82(Suppl 5): 530-535

30. Meyers SP, Wildenhain S, Chess MA, Tarr RW (1994) Postoperative evaluation for intracranial recurrence of medulloblastoma: MR findings with gadopentetate dimeglumine. AJNR 15: 1425-1434

31. Molenkamp G, Riemann B, Kuwert T, Strater R, Kurlemann G, Schober O, Jurgens H, Wolff JE (1998) Monitoring tumor activity in low grade glioma of childhood. Klin Padiatr 210: 239-242

32. Barkadjiev AI, Barnes PD, Goumnerova LC, et al. (1996) Magnetic resonance imaging changes after stereotactic radiation therapy for childhood low grade astrocytoma. Cancer 78: 864-873

33. Moringlane JR, Voges M, Huber G, et al. (1997) Short-term CT and MR changes in brain tumors following 125-I Interstitial irradiation. JCAT 21: 15-21

34. Van Tassel P, Bruner J, Moar MH, et al. (1995) MR of toxic effects of accelerated fractionation radiation therapy and carboplatin chemotherapy for malignant gliomas. AJNR 16: 715-726

35. Boyd C, Ashdown BC, Boyko O, Uglietta JP, et al. (1993) Postradiation cerebellar necrosis mimicking tumor: MR appearance. J Comput Assist Tomogr 17: 124-126

36. Torres CF, Rebsamen S, Silber JH, Sutton LN, Bilaniuk LT, Zimmerman RA, Goldwein JW, Phillips PC, Lange BJ (1994) Surveillance scanning of children with medulloblastoma. N Engl J Med 330: 892-895

37. Mendel E, Levy ML, Raffel C, McComb JG, Pikus H, Nelson MD Jr, Ganz W (1996) Surveillance imaging in children with primitive neuroectodermal tumors. Neurosurgery 38: 692-695

38. Lindsley KL (1994) Surveillance scanning of children with medulloblastoma. N Engl J Med 331: 483

39. Friedman HS (1995) More on surveillance scanning of children with medulloblastoma. N Engl J Med 332: 191

40. Steinbok P, Hentschel S, Cochrane DD, Kestle JR (1996) Value of postoperative surveillance imaging in the management of children with some common brain tumors. J Neurosurg 84: 726-732

41. Sutton LN, Cnaan A, Klatt L, Zhao H, Zimmerman R, et al. (1996) Postoperative surveillance imaging in children with cerebellar astrocytomas. J Neurosurg 84: 721-725

42. La Marca F, Tomita T (1997) Importance of patient evaluation for long-term survival in medulloblastoma recurrence. Childs Nerv Syst 13: 30-34

43. Bouffet E, Doz F, Demaille MC, et al. (1998) Improving survival in recurrent medulloblastoma: earlier detection, better treatment or still an impasse? Br J Cancer 77: 1321-1326

44. Fischbein NJ, Prados MD, Wara W, Russo C, et al. (1996) Radiologic classification of brain stem tumors: correlation of magnetic resonance imaging appearance with clinical outcome. Pediatr Neurosurg 24: 9-23

45. Smith RR, Zimmerman RA, Packer RJ, Hackney DB, et al. (1990) Pediatric brainstem glioma. Post-radiation clinical and MR follow-up. Neuroradiology 32: 265-271

Neuronal Intestinal Dysplasia and its Relation to Other Motility Disorders

W.E. Berdon

Department of Pediatric Radiology, Babies & Children's Hospital of New York, New York, USA

Introduction

During infancy at least six intestinal motility syndromes are known to occur. These are: (1) aganglionosis (Hirschsprung's disease); (2) meconium plug syndrome (also known as neonatal small left colon); (3) microcolon of prematurity; (4) CPAP belly syndrome (found in infants treated on a ventilator with continuous positive airways pressure); (5) megacystis microcolon intestinal hypoperistalsis (neonatal hollow viscus myopathy); and, (6) neuronal intestinal dysplasia.

The first five of these syndromes have diagnostic findings that either suggest or make a definite diagnosis. The sixth syndrome is a collection of failed Hirschsprung's disease and/or constipated infants or children mainly reported from Europe and Asia as having neuronal intestinal dysplasia; it is not a diagnosis made on X-ray. Current concepts on this syndrome in relation to the first five mentioned will be discussed here.

Aganglionosis (Hirschsprung's Disease)

This disease has been know for over a century. It presents with a low sigmoid colon and rectum predilection; there is strong male predominance and it is occasionally found to be familial [1, 2]. The incidence is higher in children with Down's syndrome. Cases with more extensively diseased colon (total colon, terminal ileum) are found equally among males and females. Some cases are familial and occasionally found as a syndrome with other diseases (central apnea, neuroblastoma, congenital heart disease and familial neurocristopathy).

The most commonly held theory is that cells of neural origin never developed in their appropriate place. Mutations of the *ret* gene are found in 30% of familial cases and in 15% of sporadic cases.

Meconium Plug Syndrome

This syndrome (also known as small left colon syndrome) has a high association with a previously complicated pregnancy (infant of diabetic mother, IDM, maternal $MgSO_4$). The syndrome is only rarely found to be Hirschsprung's disease. On biopsy the findings are normal.

Microcolon of Prematurity

This disease is found in premature infants weighing less than 1000 g. The infant produces no spontaneous stools. There is no relation to the type of ventilator used; however, an association with maternal $MgSO_4$ has been found. In rare cases bowel perforation occurs.

CPAP Belly

This syndrome occurs in premature infants weighing less than 1500 g who are on artificial ventilation with continuous positive airways pressure (CPAP). There is gas present from the stomach to the rectum (stem to stern).

Megacystic Microcolon-Intestinal Hypoperistalsis Syndrome

There are more ganglion cells present with this syndrome (also known as neonatal hollow viscus myopathy) than should normally be found. It is seen mainly in females. There is a huge bladder, a microcolon and non functional small intestine. Forme fruste cases occur.

Neuronal Intestinal Dysplasia: Chronic Constipation

This disease presents in two types: Type A is rare; it occurs in neonates and is caused by a congenital absence of the sympathetic chain. The symptoms are bloody diarrhea, and it is often fatal.

Type B is more common; it is found to accompany Hirschsprung's disease or can also be found alone. There is a weak correlation between clinical presentation and the extent of pathological changes. The treatment consists of enemas and laxatives.

Pruri [1] defines neuronal intestinal dysplasia as having characteristic histological findings of hyperganglionosis of the submucosal and myenteric plexus, giant ganglia, ectopic ganglia, increased acetylcholinesterase (AChE) positive fibers around the submucosal blood vessels, and increased AChE nerve fibers in L. propia.

References

1. Puri P, Ohshiro K, Wester T (1995) Hirschsprung's disease: a search for etiology. Semin Pediatr Surg 7(3): 140-148
2. Ryan DP (1995) Neuronal intestinal dysplasia. Semin Pediatr Surg 4(7): 22-25
3. Puri P, Wester T (1995) Intestinal neuronal dysplasia. Semin Pediatr Surg 7(3): 181-186
4. Scharli AF, Sossai R (1995) Hypoganglionosis. Semin Pediatr Surg 7(3): 187-191

Pathophysiology and Sonographic Correlates of Neonatal Brain Injury

G.A. Taylor

Department of Radiology, Children's Hospital and Harvard Medical School, Boston, USA

Introduction

In the last few years there have been significant advances in the understanding of the mechanisms responsible for neonatal brain injury. At the same time, ultrasound techniques have continued to improve at a dramatic pace allowing us to identify flow in sub-millimeter arteries and in the main venous drainage pathways of the brain. This presentation will review some of the new findings related to the pathophysiology of cerebrovascular injury in the newborn and how they relate to cranial sonographic findings.

Germinal Matrix Hemorrhage in the Premature

Many factors have been clinically and experimentally implicated in the pathogenesis of germinal matrix hemorrhage (GMH) [1]. Yet, despite the multiplicity of potential causes, there are two interrelated phenomena that seem to explain the development of these lesions.

The first of these processes is hypoxic ischemia, or diminished oxygen delivery to the brain. This commonly occurs under a variety of circumstances, including hypoxemia, systemic hypotension, and reduced hemoglobin concentration [1, 2]. There is increasing evidence that both the destructive processes and hemodynamic consequences of hypoxic ischemia are related to excessive synaptic accumulations of excitatory amino acids such as glutamate. In addition to inducing critically sustained cell membrane depolarization and uncontrolled neuronal autolysis [2, 3], the glutamate cascade also stimulates the production of nitric oxide by induction of the enzyme nitric oxide synthase [3]. This potent vasodilator can result in dramatic hyperemia in areas of injured brain (Fig. 1). In experimental models, a 300-400% increase in regional cerebral blood flow has been demonstrated after direct injections of micromolar concentrations of a glutamate analogue (N-methyl-d-aspartate, NMDA) [4].

There is also increasing evidence that the developing brain is particularly susceptible to excitotoxic injury. In rats for example, brain injury related to NMDA injection is 60 times greater in the neonatal animal compared to adults [5].

The second process involves alterations in cerebral hemodynamics related to extrauterine life as a sick premature. Many of the therapeutic maneuvers performed in caring for these infants have been associated with an increased risk of GMH, and appear to significantly alter intracranial venous hemodynamics (Fig. 2). Increased venous pressures have been demonstrated in infants breathing out of sequence with a mechanical ventilator, during endotracheal tube suctioning, and with high peak inspiratory pressures [1]. Other factors such tension pneumothorax, exchange transfusions, rapid infusions of colloid, and myocardial injury due to asphyxia may also have dramatic effects on venous pressures and hemodynamics [1, 6, 7].

It is likely that the combined destructive and hyperemic effects of hypoxic ischemia and therapy-related he-

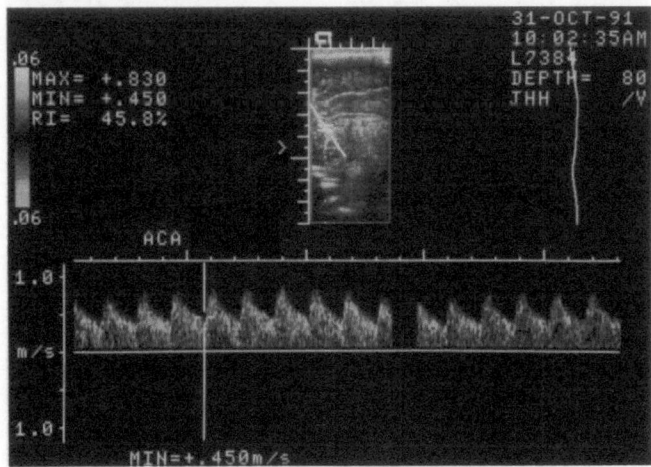

Fig. 1. Doppler waveform of anterior cerebral artery in premature infant with hypoxic ischemic injury shows markedly diminished pulsatility (RI 46%) due to increased diastolic flow consistent with cerebral hyperemia

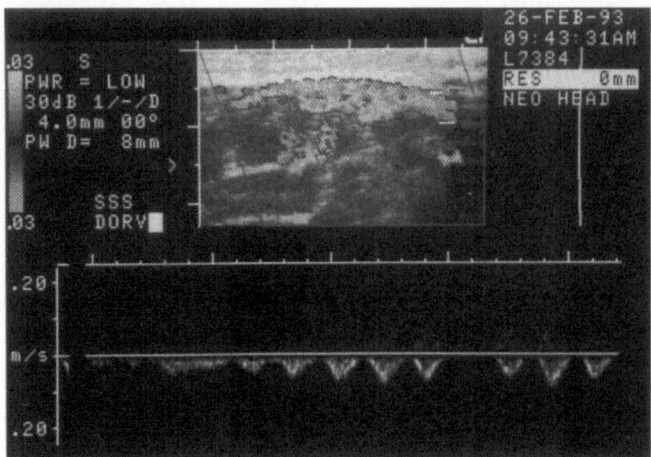

Fig. 2. Doppler waveform from superior sagittal sinus in infant with double outlet right ventricle shows increased pulsatility of venous flow caused by referred cardiac pulsations

modynamic alterations on a vulnerable vascular bed eventually lead to GMH in the premature infant.

Ghazi-Birry et al. [8] have shown that the great majority of GMH are not arterial, but venous in origin. In a detailed microscopic study of the vascular architecture

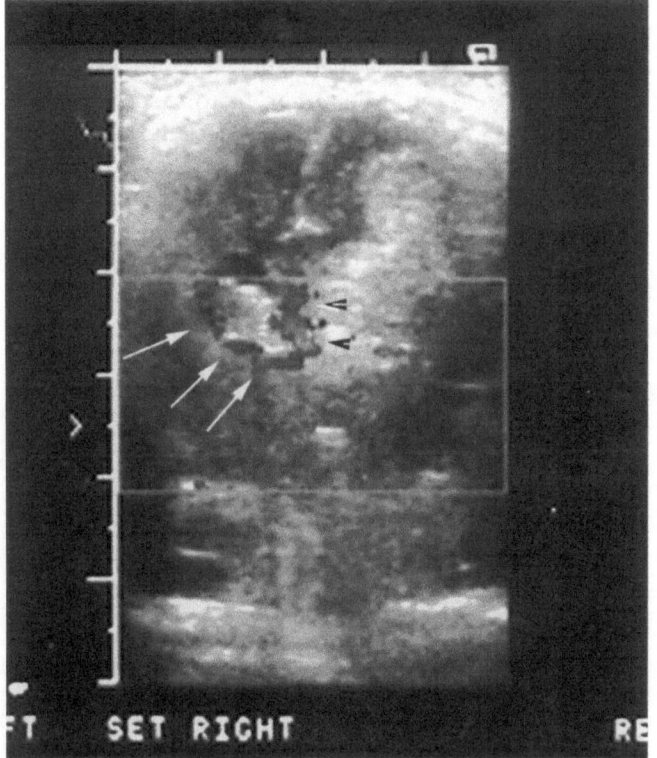

Fig. 3. Coronal color Doppler image of premature infant obtained at the level of the foramen of Monro shows bilateral germinal matrix hemorrhages and a large parenchymal on left side with obstruction of flow in the ipsilateral terminal vein. Note flow in normal contralateral teminal vein (*arrows*) and internal cerebral veins (*arrowheads*)

of the germinal matrix in premature infants with early GMH, they demonstrated tunneling of blood along perivenous spaces resulting in distortion, compression and occlusion of adjacent veins. Their findings suggest that local elevations in venous pressure within the germinal matrix play a major role in the pathophysiology of this lesion. This is important because the "cascade" of venous bleeding, perivenous leakage and distortion of larger veins appears to be the same mechanism that results in larger intraparenchymal hemorrhages. Histological studies of intraparenchymal hemorrhage as well as color Doppler ultrasound observations suggest that these hemorrhages are the result of venous infarction due to obstruction of terminal veins by large GMH (Fig. 3) [9, 10].

The principal consequences of GMH are twofold. First, is its potential for progression to more serious patterns of hemorrhage and their attendant complications such as post-hemorrhagic hydrocephalus. Second, GMH also appears to destroy neurons that originate in the germinal matrix and are destined to populate layers II to VI of the cerebral cortex [11]. This may explain some of the complex cognitive and attentional deficits seen in between 25% and 50% of premature infants [2]. Thus, the prevention of GMH continues to be an important goal.

Post-Hemorrhagic Hydrocephalus

The impairment of cerebrospinal fluid (CSF) flow during the acute phase of post-hemorrhagic hydrocephalus is thought to result from blockage of arachnoid villi and narrow ventricular passages by echogenic hemorrhagic particulate matter. Over time, the presence of blood within the ventricles and cisterns evokes an inflammatory reaction and formation of fibrous adhesions, most commonly in the cisterna magna [12, 13]. Occasionally, occlusion of both the aqueduct of Sylvius and the fourth ventricular outflow foramina may occur resulting in a "trapped", disproportionately dilated fourth ventricle [14]. The mastoid view can be helpful in identifying early or progressive dilatation of the fourth ventricle as well as other potential causes of ventricular obstruction, such as clot obstructing the 3rd or 4th ventricle (Fig. 4).

The presence of echogenic debris in the spinal subarachnoid space has been associated with progressive ventricular dilatation after severe intracranial hemorrhage or bacterial meningitis [15]. The increased echogenicity and is due to a high protein and red blood cell content in the subarachnoid space and is a marker of arachnoiditis that may help predict both the development of progressive ventricular dilatation and the failure of serial lumbar punctures as an initial therapy in infants with post-hemorrhagic or post-infectious ventricular dilatation. This finding may be helpful in identifying newborns who will not benefit from serial lumbar punctures for treatment of hydrocephalus.

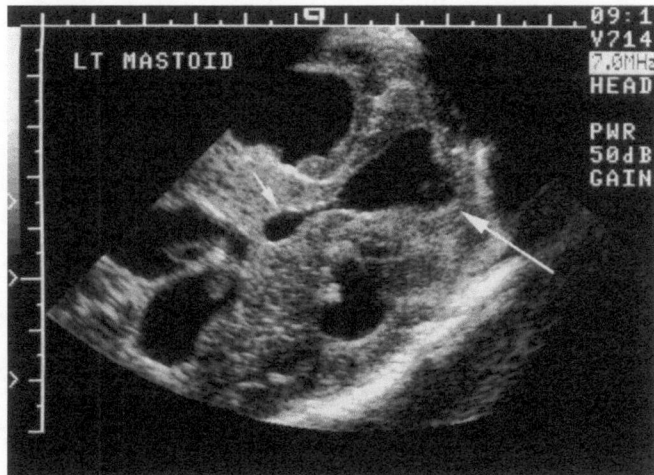

Fig. 4. Mastoid view in premature infant with post-hemorrhagic hydrocephalus shows dilated third (*small arrow*) and fourth ventricle (*large arrow*) resulting from arachnoiditis and obstruction of foramina of Luschka and Magendie. Note clot in lateral ventricles

Transcranial Doppler techniques may be used to help identify infants with elevated intracranial pressure, and to help determine the need for and optimal timing of shunt placement [16, 17].

Seibert et al. [18] have shown that an increasing resistive index (RI) correlates well with elevation in intracranial pressure (ICP) in an animal model of acute hydrocephalus. As ICP rises, arterial flow tends to be more affected during diastole than during systole, resulting in an elevated pulsatility of flow. Unfortunately, the hemodynamic response to hydrocephalus may be quite variable. Although several authors have demonstrated elevated intracranial RI in infants with hydrocephalus, and a subsequent decrease in RI after ventricular tap or shunt [19-21], other investigators have shown no difference in RI before and after treatment of hydrocephalus [22], or have shown poor correlation between RI obtained from the anterior cerebral artery and intracranial pressure [22], or considerable overlap between pre- and post-tap RI measures [23]. In addition, intracerebral artery RI in premature infants can vary widely, with values between 50 and 80 reported in normal infants less than 35 weeks' gestational age [24]. This level of variability has limited the clinical utility of intracranial Doppler in the evaluation of newborns with hydrocephalus.

The use of fontanelle compression during Doppler examination of the anterior or middle cerebral artery addresses many of these limitations and may be useful in the early identification of infants with abnormal intracranial compliance prior to the development of increased ICP as shown by elevated baseline RI [21, 25].

According to the Monro-Kellie hypothesis, the volume of brain, spinal fluid, blood and other intracranial components is constant [26]. During fontanelle compression in normal infants, CSF or blood can be readily displaced in order to compensate for the small increase in volume delivered by compression of the anterior fontanelle, resulting in no increase in ICP. As a result, the intracranial RI changes very little [25, 27]. In infants with hydrocephalus however, the increase in intracranial volume with fontanelle compression is translated into a transient increase in ICP, and an acute increase in arterial pulsatility. Serial examinations using this technique can also be used to follow an individual infant's ability to compensate for minor changes in intracranial volume and thus can be used as a noninvasive indirect measure of intracranial compliance.

In our experience, transient fontanelle compression is a safe and well-tolerated procedure, even in critically ill premature infants. Since the pressure challenges are delivered briefly (3-5 s), it is unlikely that any alterations in cerebral blood flow will be physiologically significant. However, prolonged compression of the fontanelle should be avoided. Pressure should be immediately released if heart rate significantly decreases during Doppler examination. In addition, the presence of reversed flow during diastole in a Doppler study obtained without fontanelle compression is strongly suggestive of elevated intracranial pressure, and fontanelle compression is not necessary or recommended in these patients.

References

1. Volpe JJ (1995) Intracranial hemorrhage: germinal matrix-intraventricular hemorrhage of the premature infant. In: Volpe JJ (ed) Neurology of the Newborn, 3rd edn. WB Saunders, Philadelphia, pp 403-466
2. McDonald JW, Johnston MV (1993) Excitatory amino acid neurotoxicity in the developing brain. NIDA Res Monogr 133: 185-205
3. Johnston MV, Trescher WH, Taylor GA (1995) Hypoxic and ischemic central nervous system disorders in infants and children. Adv Pediatr 42: 1-45
4. Taylor GA, Trescher WH, Johnston MV, Traystman RJ (1995) Experimental neuronal injury in the newborn lamb: a comparison of NMDA receptor blockade and nitric oxide synthesis inhibition on lesion size and cerebral hyperemia. Pediatr Res 38: 644-651
5. McDonald JW, Silverstein FS, Johnston MV(1988) Neurotoxicity of N-methyl-d-aspartate is markedly enhanced in developing rat central nervous system. Brain Res 459: 200-203
6. Perlman JM, Volpe JJ (1987) Are venous circulatory abnormalities important in the pathogenesis of hemorrhagic and/or ischemic cerebral injury? Pediatrics 80: 705-711
7. Dean LM, Taylor GA (1995) The intracranial venous system in infants: normal and abnormal findings on duplex and color Doppler sonography. AJR 164: 151-156
8. Ghazi-Birry HS, Brown WR, Moody DM, Challa VR, Block SM, Reboussin DM (1997) Venous origin of germinal matrix hemorrhage in VLBW preterm neonates and vascular characteristics of the human germinal matrix. Am J Neuroradiol 184: 219-229
9. Gould SJ, Howard S, Hope PL, Reynolds EOR (1987) Periventricular intraparenchymal cerebral hemorrhage in preterm infants: the role of venous infarction. J Pathol 151: 197-202

10. Taylor GA (1995) Effect of germinal matrix hemorrhage on terminal vein position and patency. Pediatr Radiol 25: S37-S40
11. Volpe JJ (1996) Subplate neurons, missing link in brain injury of the premature brain? Pediatrics 1: 112-113
12. De Vries LS, Larroche J-C, Levene MI (1988) Intracranial sequelae. In: Levene MI, Bennett MJ, Punt J (eds) Fetal and neonatal neurology and neurosurgery. Churchill-Livingstone, New York, pp 346-353
13. Gurtner P, Bass T, Gudeman SK, et al. (1992) Surgical management of posthemorrhagic hydrocephalus in 22 low-birth-weight infants. Nerv Syst 8: 198-202
14. Hall TR, Choi A, Schellinger D, et al. (1992) Isolation of the fourth ventricle causing transtentorial herniation: neurosonographic findings in premature infants. AJR 159: 811-815
15. Rudas G, Almássy Z, Papp B, Varga E, Méder Ü, Taylor GA (1998) Echodense spinal subarachnoid space in neonates with progressive ventricular dilatation: a marker of noncommunicating hydrocephalus. AJR 171: 1119-1121
16. Chadduck WM, Seibert JJ (1989) Intracranial duplex Doppler; practical uses in pediatric neurology and neurosurgery. J Child Neurol 4: S77-S86
17. Lui K, Hellman J, Sprigg A, et al. (1990) Cerebral blood-flow velocity patterns in post-hemorrhagic ventricular dilatation. Childs Nerv Syst 6: 250-253
18. Seibert JJ, McCowan TC, Chadduck WM, et al. (1989) Duplex pulsed Doppler US versus intracranial pressure in the neonate: clinical and experimental studies. Radiology 171: 155-159
19. Taylor GA, Short LB, Walker LK, et al. (1990) Intracranial blood flow: quantification with duplex Doppler and color Doppler flow US. Radiology 176: 231-236
20. Volpe JJ (1995) Intracranial hemorrhage: germinal matrix-intraventricular hemorrhage of the premature infant. In: Volpe JJ (ed) Neurology of the newborn, 3rd edn. WB Saunders, Philadelphia, pp 403-463
21. Taylor GA, Phillips MD, Ichord RN, et al. (1994) Doppler evaluation of intracranial compliance in infants. Radiology 191: 787-791
22. Goh D, Minns RA, Hendry GMA, et al. (1992) Cerebrovascular resistive index assessed by duplex Doppler sonography and its relationship to intracranial pressure in infantile hydrocephalus. Pediatr Radiol 22: 246-250
23. Goh D, Minns RA, Pye SD, et al. (1991) Cerebral blood flow velocity changes after ventricular taps and ventriculoperitoneal shunting. Childs Nerv Syst 7: 452-457
24. Horgan JG, Rumack CM, Hay T, et al. (1989) Absolute intracranial blood-flow velocities evaluated by duplex Doppler sonography in asymptomatic preterm and term neonates. AJR 152: 1059-1064
25. Taylor GA, Madsen JR (1996) Neonatal hydrocephalus hemodynamic response to fontanelle compression: correlation with intracranial pressure and need for shunt placement. Radiology 201: 685-689
26. Bruce DA, Berman WA, Schut L (1977) Cerebrospinal fluid pressure monitoring in children: physiology, pathology and clinical usefulness. Adv Pediatr 24: 233-290
27. Taylor GA (1992) Effect of scanning pressure on intracranial hemodynamics during transfontanellar duplex Doppler examinations. Radiology 185: 763-766

Imaging Tumor Angiogenesis Using Contrast-Enhanced Magnetic Resonance Imaging

R.C. Brasch

Contrast Media Laboratory and Center for Pediatric Pharmaceutical and Molecular Imaging, Department of Radiology
University of California, San Francisco, USA

Introduction

Magnetic resonance imaging (MRI) enhanced with contrast media has the potential to measure the level of angiogenesis in cancers and to monitor the immediate effects of drugs intended to inhibit angiogenesis. To appreciate the significance of such potential, it is necessary to first understand what is angiogenesis and why it is receiving so much attention.

Angiogenesis is the process by which new vessels grow toward and into a tissue. The angiogenesis process is required for normal physiologic processes including embryogenesis, corpus luteum formation, and wound healing. It is also a critical element in the pathogenesis of several disease processes, most notably rapid growth and metastasis of solid tumors. With the recent emergence of new interventional strategies and drugs to halt in the angiogenesis process, the need to understand angiogenesis has emerged from the realm of the laboratory to clinical practice.

The formation of new blood supply is essential to the unrestricted growth of tumors. Tumors do not produce their own new blood vessels (with the exception of hemangioendotheliomas), but for nutrients and oxygen must rely on vascular supply derived from the nearby host tissue. Judah Folkman, a pediatric surgeon and a recognized pioneer in the investigation of angiogenesis, has shown that tumors can attain a size of only 1-2 mm by simple diffusion of nutrients, but can exist for an extended period in this quiescent, static-sized, prevascular stage before angiogenesis is "switched on" [1]. Once angiogenesis is upregulated, the tumor enters the vascular phase allowing for exponential growth and resultant clinical manifestations. Many laboratories are attempting to precisely identify and characterize "the angiogenesis switch", the triggering mechanism by which a small nest of neoplastic cells can take on malignant growth characteristics and metastasize. Once *switched on*, angiogenic factors elaborated by the tumor and tumor-associated inflammatory cells, sometimes referred to as signaling molecules, interact with endothelial cells in neighboring vessels to stimulate new capillary buds and to prepare the local environment for their ingrowth.

The potential of a tumor to successfully metastasize has also been linked to angiogenesis, neovasculature being required at both the beginning and the end of the metastatic cascade. More angiogenic primary tumors possess a greater number and size of microvessels through which the metastasizing cells are shed into the bloodstream; with increased angiogenesis the number of metastasizing cells can increase 100-fold [2]. The well-recognized hyperpermeability of tumor vessels, a pathophysiologic trait directly tied to angiogenesis, may also contribute to the transendothelial escape of tumor cells [3]; new proliferating capillaries have fragmented [3] basement membranes and widened interendothelial gaps that probably account for this hyperpermeability. Having entered the circulation, the metastasizing cells must survive the journey, escape immune surveillance, penetrate (or grow from within) the microvessels of the target organ, and again induce angiogenesis at the target in order to grow beyond 2 mm in diameter. It should be noted that angiogenesis may not be sufficient, in itself, for metastases to occur. However, the inhibition of angiogenesis prevents the growth of tumor cells at both the primary and secondary sites and thereby can prevent the emergence of metastases [4].

Recognizing angiogenesis as a limiting factor for both tumor growth and metastases, it has been postulated that angiogenesis correlates with tumor aggressiveness. Indeed, this assumption has been supported in numerous clinical series investigating a variety of tumor types. Histologic assays of angiogenesis based on the microvascular density (MVD) (the number of endothelial cell clusters counted in a high-power microscopic field), in randomly selected human cancers showed that MVD correlated, as an independent factor, with the presence of metastases at time of diagnosis and with decreased patient survival times [5, 6]. In other words, if the angiogenic status of a tumor can be measured, then an important determinant of tumor biology and patient outcome, independent of the tumor cell type, can be measured. In recent years, the adverse prognostic significance of a high histologic MVD, measured by the pathologist, has

Table 1. Human malignancies for which histologic microvascular density (MVD) has correlated with local aggressiveness, metastatic rate, and/or adverse prognosis [6]

Breast carcinoma
Lung carcinoma
Prostate carcinoma
Head and neck (squamous) carcinoma
Rectum carcinoma
Testicle carcinoma
Bladder carcinoma
Ovary carcinoma
Soft tissue tumors
Central nervous system tumors
Multiple myeloma

been demonstrated in a wide range of human cancers (Table 1) and is often used as the most easily measured surrogate of angiogenesis.

Angiogenesis is a complex process with interactions of both promoters and inhibitors in a system of checks and balances. Normally quiescent with remarkably slow rates of cell turnover, endothelial cells can rapidly proliferate and form new blood vessels in response to a net positive balance of angiogenic factors [7]. Promoters, termed "angiogenic factors", are produced by neoplastic cells and tumor-associated inflammatory cells and act locally in a paracrine fashion to increase the production of endothelial cells and to prepare the local environment for the ingrowth of new vascular buds. Some of the recognized angiogenesis promoters are listed in Table 2. Under the influence of these chemical signaling molecules, endothelial cells in tumor blood vessels divide rapidly, whereas those in normal tissues do not [7].

Vascular endothelial growth factor, also know as vascular permeability factor (VEGF/VPF) has been studied extensively and is an appealing target for angiogenesis intervention. This peptide stimulator is expressed by many cancer types and is not only mitogenic for endothelial cells (hence, the origin for one of its names, VEGF) but also induces dramatic increases in vascular permeability (a property expressed in its other name, VPF) to macromolecules, including serum proteins. Apparently, the release of VEGF/VPF from tumor cells induces hyperpermeability in nearby capillaries, leading

Table 2. Endogenous stimulators of angiogenesis

Acidic fibroblastic growth factor (aFGF)
Angiogenin
Basic fibroblastic growth factor (bFGF)
Heparinase
Interleukin-8
Placenta growth factor
Platelet-derived endothelial cell growth factor
Prostaglandins E_1, E_2
Tumor necrosis factor alpha
Vascular endothelial growth factor/vascular permeability factor
   (VEGF/VPF)

to the oozing of proteinaceous fluid into the paratumoral interstitial space. A proteinaceous gel forms providing an ideal matrix for the ingrowth of new capillary buds. Thus, VEGF/VPF is involved in an early stage of the angiogenesis cascade, in tissue preparation for the development of new capillaries.

Of importance to diagnostic imagers, the VEGF/VPF-induced hyperpermeability to macromolecules provides a window of opportunity for an imaging assay of the angiogenesis process. It should be noted that the increase in permeability of cancer microvessels has always been demonstrated with large molecules (greater than 30 000 Da), and has not been shown with small molecular probes such as inulin (approximately 1000 Da), or with small molecular gadolinium contrast media (about 600 Da). The size of the molecule is thus of critical importance in the design of an imaging strategy for detecting and measuring up-regulated angiogenesis.

Progress in the Imaging of Angiogenesis

Although microscopic counting of capillaries on immunohistochemically stained tumor specimens has been a useful surrogate of angiogenesis, MVD is not a "gold standard" of angiogenesis nor is it an ideal clinical tool. By requiring a tissue biopsy, at the minimum, serial MVD assays to monitor progress of therapy is not practical. Histologic MVD is also subject to sampling errors because tumors are notoriously heterogeneous and the entire tumor cannot be examined, only 10 µm-thick slices that may not contain the most angiogenically active tumor portions. Clearly an imaging assay for angiogenic activity would be welcome and should be clinically powerful, particularly if the method was quantitative, non-invasive, could sample the entire tumor, and could be repeated at frequent intervals.

In a qualitative way, radiologists have been imaging tumor angiogenesis for decades, we have called it "vascularity" and have commented on its relative density on the "capillary phase" of angiograms. The typical hypervascularity of cancers may be largely responsible for the high sensitivity of gadopentetate-enhanced MRI for the detection of breast cancers [8]; the dense microvascular network of cancers leads to a higher tumor accumulation of contrast medium than in normal breast tissue, even though the small-molecular (~600 Da) contrast medium rapidly diffuses through the capillary walls of both normal and tumor vessels.

Macromolecular contrast media (MMCM), now being developed for both MRI and CT, have molecular sizes that approximate the size of serum proteins, or larger, and are thus well suited to define the hypervascularity and hyperpermeability of cancer microvessels [9-13]. These MMCM diffuse very slowly, if at all, through normal endothelial barriers. Although not yet in clinical use, several contrast media manufacturers and

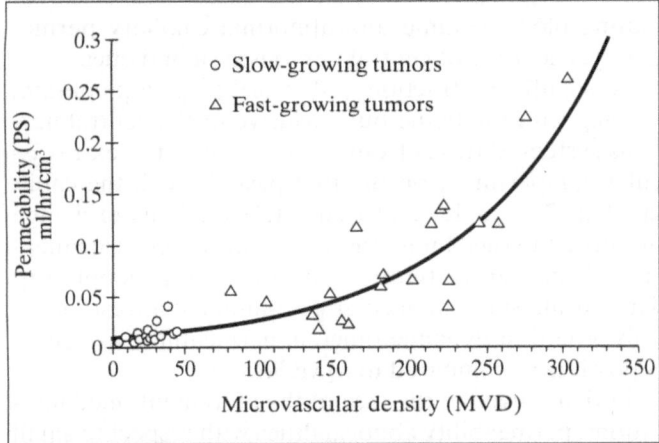

Fig. 1. Scatter plot of values for permeability surface area products (PS), derived from dynamic MMCM-enhanced MRI, for both slow growing (o) and fast growing (Δ) adenocarcinomas shows a close correlation ($r = 0.80$) with histologic microvascular densities (MVD). The log-transformed fit is superimposed. Note that both MRI and histologic techniques can differentiate the two types of tumors and that permeabilities seem to increase exponentially with microvascular density, and thus with angiogenesis. (Modified from and reproduced with permission of *Radiology*) [10]

research laboratories are working to select suitable formulations for advanced clinical development. In addition to characterizing microvessels, MMCM can be used advantageously for large vessel angiography as these macromolecules recirculate in the blood for 1 h or longer; angiograms can be obtained both before and after an intervention or in multiple anatomic regions, but with only a single contrast medium administration. Quantitative measurements of tissue blood volume and permeability, expressed respectively as the fractional blood volume (fBV) and as the permeability surface area product (PS) may emerge as the most valuable gain from MMCM [14-16]. Our group has reported that using a prototype MMCM, albumin-(Gd-DTPA)$_{35}$, MRI of experimental mammary adenocarcinomas provided estimates of tumor blood volumes and microvascular permeabilities (PS) that correlated strongly ($r^2 - 0.80$) with histologic measurements of MVD (Fig. 1) [10].

The two mammary tumor types studied, one slow-growing and the other fast and aggressive, could be differentiated and graded by MRI with respect to their angiogenic profiles. The MRI estimates of permeability with respect to the macromolecular contrast agent was particularly well correlated with the histologic assay of angiogenesis and PS was statistically ($p<0.01$) higher in the more aggressive tumor subgroup.

The MRI characterization of microvascularity offers certain advantages over the histologic assay because MRI is noninvasive, is able to sample the entire tumor, can be repeated frequently to monitor the effect of therapy, and reflects both the anatomy (vascular volume) and the physiology of the tumor (permeability).

Additional studies were undertaken by our group to determine whether MMCM-enhanced MRI could identify and measure the effect of an anti-angiogenesis intervention on tumor microvessels. The effects of monoclonal anti-VEGF antibody, generated as a pharmaceutical by recombinant DNA methodology, on MRI microvascular characteristics and on tumor growth were examined in a human breast cancer model, MDA-MB-435, implanted in athymic rats. Administration of the anti-VEGF antibody (three 1 mg doses at 3-day intervals or a single 1 mg dose) induced significant reductions in both tumor growth rate after 1 week of treatment ($p<0.05$) and in MRI-assayed permeability ($p<0.05$). The effect of anti-VEGF antibody on the tumor microvessels could be observed as early as 30 min after antibody administration and the effect was not subtle (Fig. 2). Consider the implications of monitoring the effectiveness of angiogenesis inhibition in 1 h or even 1 day, compared to the usual 4-6 week wait we now tolerate to monitor potential changes in tumor volume.

These results confirm that new microvessels formed in response to angiogenesis are hyperpermeable to macromolecules and that hyperpermeability is a mechanistic element in angiogenesis. This ability to measure variations in tumor-vessel hyperpermeability should be useful to assess anti-angiogenesis therapy.

A variety of contrast-enhanced MRI and analytical techniques have been proposed for the characterization of tumors [8, 17-23]. However, in addition to using a macromolecular contrast agent, our technique has some additional unique features. It utilizes a 3-dimensional spoiled gradient recalled echo (SPGR) data acquisition that permits broad anatomic multislice coverage of the entire tumor and eliminates inflow signal misregistration in vessels within the central sections, a necessity for

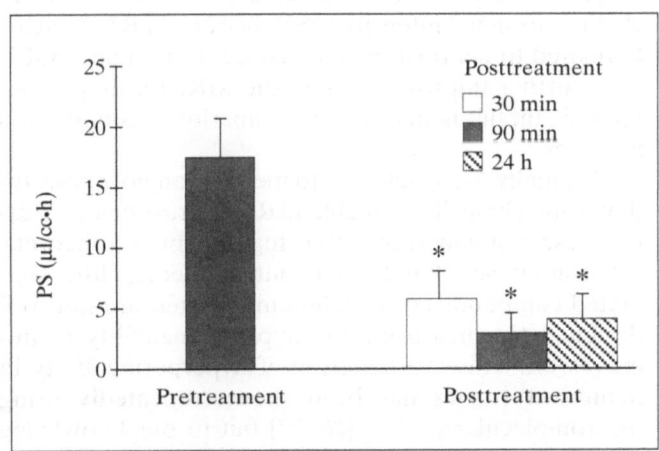

Fig. 2. Histogram of permeability surface products (PS) in a human breast tumor model estimated from dynamic MRI enhanced with a macromolecular contrast medium (MMCM), albumin-(Gd-DTPA)$_{35}$, before and at 30 min, 90 min and 24 h after a single i.p. 1 mg dose of anti-VEGF antibody
*significant ($p<0.05$) differences from precontrast values

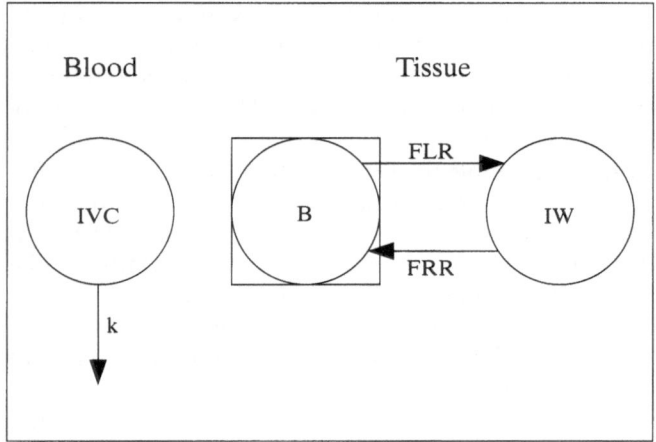

Fig. 3. Diagram of linear two-compartment model defining the fractional leak rate (FLR) of albumin-(Gd-DTPA)$_{35}$ from the vascular compartment (B) into the interstitial water (IW) and the fractional reflux rate (FRR) from the interstitial water back into the vascular space in a target tissue. The magnetic resonance signal response from the vascular space of the tumor tissue is assumed to have the same temporal form as that in a slow-moving venous structure, the IVC. The temporal loss of contrast enhancement in the IVC is described by simple monoexponential decay behavior, reflected in the decay constant, k

monitoring signal intensity responses of blood. We have also chosen an established two-compartment kinetic model of permeability which considers movement of contrast medium both into and out from the tumor interstitium [24, 25] (Fig. 3). Potential variations in the input function, blood contrast medium concentration, can be anticipated with inter-subject variations in injection rates and blood clearance, but responses in blood signal intensity are monitored in this technique in parallel with target tissue responses to correct for such variations. Changes in longitudinal relaxation rates (Δ R1) are measured and used in the kinetic analyses, in preference to changes in signal intensity (ΔSI), because Δ R1 is linearly related to contrast medium concentration and ΔSI is not. Further improvements in the MRI technique and analysis methods may provide superior feasibility and accuracy.

Optimally, we would like to measure angiogenesis today using clinically available MRI contrast media. Further research may show this is feasible, but on theoretical grounds, small molecular contrast media, either iodinated compounds or gadolinium chelates, are not well designed for measuring the hyperpermeability of microvessels. This characteristic of hyperpermeability in malignant tissues has been shown repeatedly using macromolecular probes [26, 27] but to our knowledge has not been shown for molecules smaller than 1000 Da. It is noteworthy that gadopentetate and similar small molecular contrast media quickly equilibrate between the intravascular and interstitial spaces. Due to this high vascular extraction rate, even in normal microvessels, small molecules have inherent disadvantages for esti-

mating blood volume and abnormal capillary permeability, exclusive of central nervous system tissues.

A significant fraction (10-70%) of gadopentetate, varying with the tissue but exclusive of the central nervous system, diffuses from the blood into the extravascular compartment on the first pass through the capillary bed. This rapid and variable transcapillary exchange in normal tissues limits the potential to detect or measure hyperpermeability associated with neoplasms. Thus, using small molecular gadolinium contrast media only a modest dynamic range in permeability measures is possible as compared to MMCM.

Perhaps, even in the face of the aforementioned limitations, permeability abnormalities with respect to small molecular probes will follow the pattern of macromolecules. Carefully controlled comparisons of small molecular and macromolecular contrast media for tumor characterization are needed. Alternatively, we may have to await the clinical development and governmental approval of macromolecular contrast media before these quantitative microvascular characterizations can be performed in patients. With either scenario, one can envision the frequent request from clinicians for MRI examinations to "grade the angiogenesis" of newly diagnosed tumors and to follow the progress of tumor therapy, particularly with the new generation of anti-angiogenesis interventions.

References

1. Folkman J (1989) What is the evidence that tumors are angiogenesis dependent? J Natl Cancer Inst 82: 4-6
2. Liotta LA, Kleinerman J, Saidel GM (1974) Quantitative relationships of intravascular tumor cells, tumor vessels and pulmonary metastases following tumor implantation. Cancer Res 34: 997-1004
3. Jain R, Gerlowski L (1984) Extravascular transport in normal and tumor tissues. Crit Rev Oncol Hematol 5: 115-170
4. Fidler I, Ellis L (1994) The implication of angiogenesis for the biology and therapy of cancer metastases. Cell 79: 185-188
5. Weidner N, Semple J, Welch W, Folkman J (1991) Tumor angiogensis and metasasis: correlation in invasive breast carcinoma. N Engl J Med 324: 1-8
6. Weidner N (1995) Intratumoral microvascular density as a prognostic factor in cancer. Am J Pathol 147: 9-19
7. Folkman J (1992) Introduction: angiogenesis and cancer. Semin Cancer Biol 3: 47-48
8. Heywang-Köbrunner S (1994) Contrast-enhanced magnetic resonance imaging of the breast. Invest Radiol 29: 94-104
9. Aicher KP, Dupon JW, White DL, et al. (1990) Contrast-enhanced magnetic resonance imaging of tumor-bearing mice treated with human recombinant tumor necrosis factor alpha. Cancer Res 50: 7376-7381
10. van Dijke C, Brasch R, Roberts T, et al. (1996) Mammary carcinoma model: correlation of macromolecular contrast enhanced MR imaging characterizations of tumor microvasculature and histologic capillary density. Radiology 198: 813-818
11. Schwickert H, Stiskal M, Roberts T, et al. (1996) Contrast-enhanced MRI assessment of tumor capillary permeability: the effect of pre-irradiation on the tumor delivery of chemotherapy. Radiology 198: 893-898

12. Cohen F, Kuwatsuru R, Shames D, et al. (1995) Contrast enhanced MRI estimation of altered capillary permeability in experimental mammary carcinomas following irradiation. Invest Radiol 29: 970-977
13. Daldrup H, Shames D, Wendland M, et al. (1998) Correlation of dynamic contrast-enhanced magnetic resonance imaging with histologic tumor grade: comparison of macromolecular and small molecular contrast media. Am J Roentgen 171: 941-949
14. Schmiedl U, Ogan MD, Paajanen H, et al. (1987) Albumin labeled with Gd-DTPA as an intravascular, blood pool-enhancing agent for MR imaging: biodistribution and imaging studies. Radiology 162: 205-210
15. Kuwatsuru R, Shames D, Mühler A, et al. (1993) Quantification of tissue plasma volume in the rat by contrast-enhanced magnetic resonance imaging. Magn Reson Med 30: 76-81
16. Schwickert H, Stiskal M, van Dijke C, et al. (1995) Tumor angiography using high resolution 3D MRI: comparison of Gd-DTPA and a macromolecular blood pool contrast agent. Acad Radiol 2: 851-858
17. Kaiser W, Zeitler E (1989) MR imaging of the breast: fast imaging sequences with and without Gd-DTPA. Radiology 170: 681-686
18. Stack JP, Redmond OM, Codd MB, Dervan PA, Ennis JT (1990) Breast disease: tissue characterization with Gd-DTPA enhancement profiles. Radiology 174: 491-494
19. Buadu L, Murakami J, Murayama S, Hashiguchi N, Masuda K, Toyoshima S (1996) Correlation between contrast-enhanced MR imaging of the breast and tumor angiogenesis: a quantitative and qualitative study. In: Annual Meeting American Roengen Ray Society. San Diego, Abstract 58
20. Tofts P, Berkowitz B, Schnall M (1995) Quantitative analysis of dynamic Gd-DTPA enhancement in breast tumors using a permeability model. Magn Reson Med 33: 564-568
21. Stomper P, Herman S, Klippenstein D, et al. (1995) Suspect breast lesions: findings at dynamic gadolinium-enhanced MR imaging correlated with mammographic and pathologic features. Radiology 197: 387-395
22. Weinreb J, Newstead G (1995) MR imaging of the breast. Radiology 196: 593-610
23. Spraggins T, de Paredes E, DeAngelis G (1993) Three-dimensional keyhole imaging: application to dynamic contrast-enhanced MRI of the breast. Proceedings of the Society of Magnetic Resonance in Medicine. Berkeley, Abstract 115
24. Renkin EM (1959) Transport of potassium-42 from blood to tissue in isolated mammalian skeletal muscles. Am J Physiol 197: 1205-1210
25. Crone C (1963) The permeability of capillaries in various organs determined by the use of the "indicator diffusion" method. Acta Physiol Scand 58: 292-305
26. Jain R (1987) Transport of molecules across tumor vasculature. Cancer Metastasis Rev 6: 559-593
27. Gerlowski LE, Jain RK (1986) Microvascular permeability of normal and neoplastic tissues. Microvasc Res 31: 288-305

SESSION III

SESSION III

Imaging Follow-up of Bone Neoplasia

P. Babyn

Department of Diagnostic Imaging, Hospital for Sick Children, University of Toronto, Toronto, Canada

Introduction

Imaging plays a vital role not only in initial diagnosis and staging of malignant bone tumors but also during therapy where it offers insights into pre-surgical chemotherapeutic response and post-surgical recurrence. Imaging is used following surgery or radiation to demonstrate tumor recurrence and surgical complications, which are especially common following limb-salvage surgery (LSS).

This review focuses on malignant bone sarcomas primarily osteogenic, and Ewing's sarcomas, as these are the two most commonly encountered malignant bone tumors in children, most often arising in the lower extremities [1-4]. With the advent of the newer imaging modalities and combined therapies now available, patient survival has increased dramatically over the last two decades. Radiologists need to be aware of the current treatment protocols for pediatric bone sarcomas and the effects of chemotherapy, surgery and radiation on tumor appearance.

Current Treatment Protocols

The choice of therapy for osteogenic and Ewing's sarcomas depends on a number of factors including tumor type, site of tumor origin, local extension, the presence or absence of regional and distant metastases, grade of malignancy, and response to neoadjuvant therapy. Historically amputation was the primary therapeutic option. Now however this debilitating surgical procedure is usually replaced by a combination of neoadjuvant and adjuvant chemotherapy, local resection and reconstructive surgery with or without radiation.

Treatment regimens using neoadjuvant and/or adjuvant chemotherapy have significantly improved prognosis and led to a relapse-free survival rate of about 60% [5]. Systemic multi-agent (neoadjuvant) chemotherapy given before surgery aims to eradicate potential micrometastases and reduce primary tumor size allowing improved preoperative tumor demarcation and more limited surgery [6].

Limb-salvage surgery (LSS) has become the most widely used and surgically accepted method to treat these malignancies [7, 8]. It is estimated that 80% of solitary bone malignancies are now treated by LSS in most large centers [9]. Evidence suggests that LSS offers excellent local tumor control with the advantage of preservation of function. The local recurrence and survival rates of the patients treated with LSS and amputation are comparable [10].

Evaluating Response to Chemotherapy

The degree of tumor response to neoadjuvant chemotherapy is an important prognostic factor associated with local control and long-term survival [11]. Histologic evaluation of chemotherapy response at the time of surgery remains the most definitive way to assess chemotherapy response. More than 90% tumor cell necrosis at the time of surgery indicates a good response. In poor respondents with less than 90% tumor necrosis in resected specimens, there is an increased likelihood of tumor progression and death [12].

If accurate presurgical evaluation of response to chemotherapy with imaging were possible it could have a significant impact on the choice and timing of neoadjuvant chemotherapy, patient selection for LSS and planning of radiation therapy. The benefits of individualizing chemotherapy for patients include potential reduction of therapy-related morbidity and mortality, optimizing the timing of surgical intervention and optimizing use of neo-adjuvant presurgical and postsurgical adjuvant chemotherapy. However, currently most patients with bone tumors are treated with standardized trial protocols with little opportunity for individualization [6].

Clinical evaluation of tumor response following chemotherapy using biochemical markers or subjective evaluation of local pain and warmth is not reliable. Conventional radiographs and static imaging of tumor size with computed tomography (CT) and magnetic resonance (MR) or sonography are also poor at determining tumor response. Evaluating tumor size alone is often unreliable in predicting histologic response as it may be influenced by edema, hemorrhage, or other secondary events and even massive tumor necrosis may not respond with decreased tumor bulk [13].

In osteosarcoma, no change or an increase in tumor volume and an increase in bone destruction tends to indicate a poor response to chemotherapy. A satisfactory treatment response is generally marked by decreased tumor bulk, in combination with increased calcification of the soft tissue osteoid and increased periosteal reactive bone. In Ewing's, with a good chemotherapeutic response, one tends to see disappearance of the soft tissue mass, solidification of periosteal reaction, reconstitution of cortical bone and development of coarse trabeculation within the bone [11, 14]. In Ewing's indicators of a poor chemotherapeutic response include a residual or increased soft tissue mass, and interruption or a lack of healing response [6].

The role of skeletal scintigraphy in monitoring chemotherapy is controversial as increased activity may reflect tumor healing with medullary reactive bone formation, periosteal new bone, previous fracture or residual tumor. Although not routinely used clinically, changes in TcS^{99m} plasma clearance levels have been used to define good and poor respondents. After chemotherapy regional plasma clearance decreased substantially in good respondents. Other radionuclides including thallium-^{201} and FDG and position emission tomography scanning have been used and found helpful in preliminary studies. A significant reduction in uptake of thallium-^{201} after chemotherapy indicates a favorable response [6].

Sonography has been used to monitor the effect of preoperative chemotherapy both by assessing extra-osseous tumor size and tumor flow [13, 14]. It is limited in assessment of intra-osseous tumor and cannot reliably distinguish between viable and necrotic tumor [14]. Sequential Color Doppler sonography can be used to examine extra-osseous tumor blood flow especially in the extremities. Before chemotherapy the resistive indices were significantly lower than the contralateral extremity flow. Histopathologic response could be predicted after the second course of chemotherapy with persistent decreased resistive indices present in poor responders [14].

Magnetic Resonance

Magnetic Resonance (MR) is now considered the most reliable imaging modality for tumor staging preoperatively and can be used to monitor response to chemotherapy especially with dynamic imaging [15]. It is important to realize that chemotherapy may change the signal intensity on MR of adjacent tissues and not just the underlying tumor. For example hematopoietic growth factors are often given to increase normal hematopoiesis in patients on chemotherapy and reduce the risk of infection. These factors lead to increased hematopoietic marrow being present that is readily evident with MR. This may alter the appearance of normal marrow adjacent to the tumor from normal fatty marrow to a more vascular hematopoietic marrow, and can decrease the tumor to normal marrow contrast especially on T1-weighted imaging.

With Ewing's sarcoma, residual high signal on T2-weighted imaging may not necessarily represent a poor tumor response. The St. Jude's group has shown that Ewing's may show increased signal intensity even with a good tumor response. They correlated this to an increase in interstitial fluid and decrease in the lipid cytoplasm of yellow marrow [11]. Other causes of high signal include hemorrhage and fibroblastic reactive tissue [11].

Dynamic enhanced imaging on MR is a promising new technique with a stated accuracy of more than 90% in predicting tumor response histologically [11]. This is a functional technique that provides additional information to the static determination of changes in tumor volume. Utilizing rapid sequential imaging following a bolus injection of contrast, changes in the rate of tumor enhancement are obtained. These methods have been automated allowing calculation of dynamic vector magnitude, a function of the initial rate of contrast accumulation and maximum enhancement and other factors.

Radiation Therapy

Radiation therapy is occasionally used in treatment of unresected Ewing's sarcomas. Following radiation, changes in the affected bone may be evident for several years with gradual healing. The subsequent appearance of a lytic area within the irradiated region is suspicious for local tumor recurrence or development of a second malignancy. On T2-weighted images high signal intensity may be noted from residual or recurrent tumor or from radiation induced necrosis. A decrease in marrow signal intensity after chemotherapy may be seen with tumor recurrence [11].

Amputation and Limb-Salvage Surgery

Amputation may be required when wide surgical margins are not achievable or an effective reconstructive method is not available. Amputation may also be necessary with involvement of the neurovascular bundle or tumor progression on chemotherapy.

Limb-salvage surgery (LSS) refers to a variety of different surgerical procedures, which are often individualized to the specific clinical problem at hand. LSS includes insertion of allografts, free vascularized autografts, allograft-endoprosthesis composites, massive endoprosthesis placement, Van-Nes rotationplasty, and resection arthrodesis [16-18]. LSS offers an improved functional outcome over amputation. There are a wide variety of prosthetic components now available for reconstruction including some that will allow for future

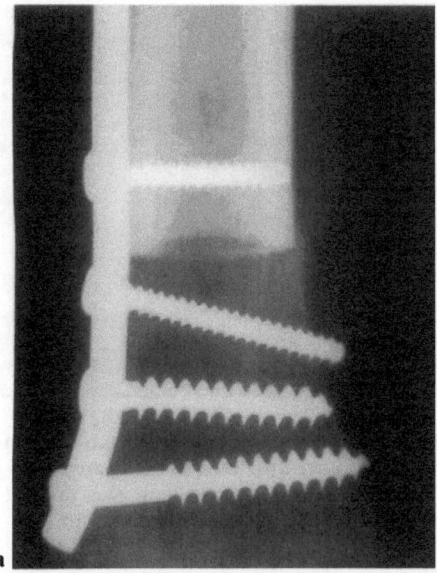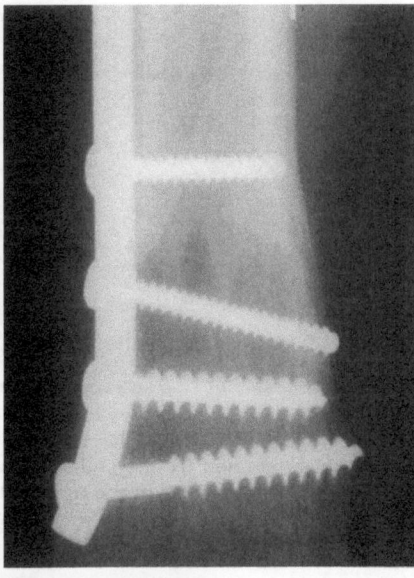

Fig. 1 a, b. Plain X-rays obtained from a child with femoral allograft. **a** Radiograph obtained shortly after surgery. **b** Radiograph obtained 16 months after the surgery shows allograft incorporation

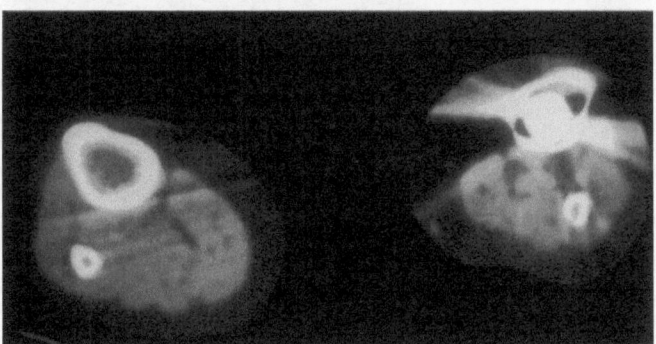

Fig. 2. Transaxial leg CT scan obtained from a child with infected endoprosthesis (the same patient as in Fig. 7) shows metallic artifact degrading the image

erative appearance. With insertion of an allograft, fusion of the allograft to adjacent native bone should occur within 1 year (Fig. 1). Myositis ossificans may occur and is usually seen early on. Occasionally one may see lucency at the graft-cement interface representing active resorption, bone remodeling or, when more extensive, aseptic loosening.

Cadaver allografts can have a variable MR imaging appearance that may simulate recurrent disease or complications [11]. Low T1 and high T2 weighted signal may be seen in keeping with necrosis. On CT and MR extensive artifact can be seen with metallic endoprostheses (Fig. 2). This artifact can be minimized with short echo pulse sequences and other specifically designed sequences [11].

growth of the extremity with expansile components. As the number of patients undergoing LSS increases, it is clear that this patient population will require numerous surgical revisions due to prosthetic failure, fractures and other complications or intervening growth.

It is important to know the normal expected post-op-

Complications Following Limb Salvage

Following LSS fractures are the most common complications seen most often in patients with allograft. All cases of post LSS fractures seen in our institution were diagnosed on plain radiographs (Fig. 3). Most fractures occur in the

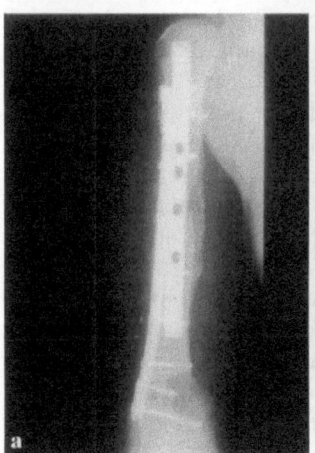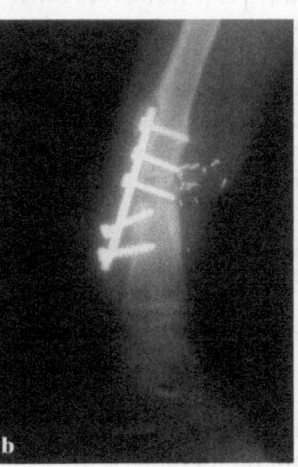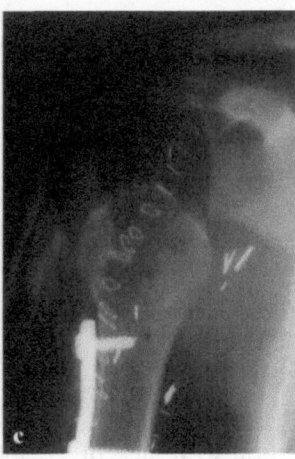

Fig. 3. a Plain X-ray obtained from a child with a right humeral allograft shows a fracture in the midshaft of the allograft. The fracture was fixed with a side plate and multiple screws. **b** Plain X-ray obtained from a child with a van-Nes rotationplasty shows delayed union. There were displacement of the van-Nes graft and failure of the screws. **c** Plain X-ray obtained from a child (same patient as in **a** shows joint subluxation of the right humeral allograft

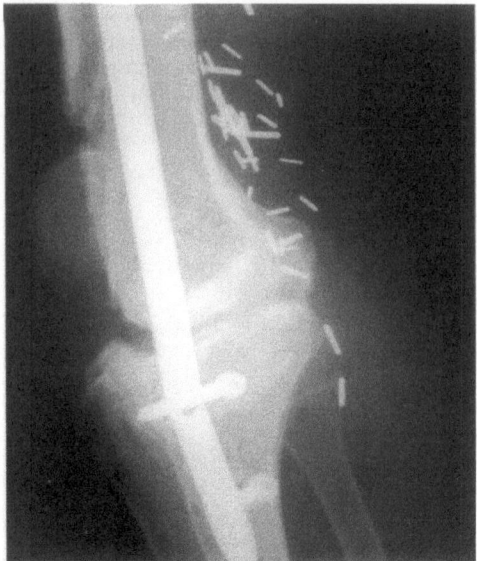

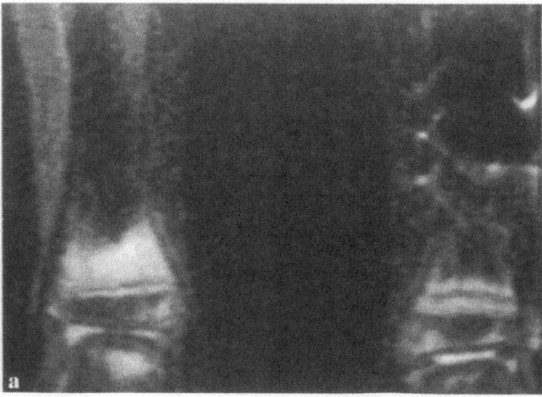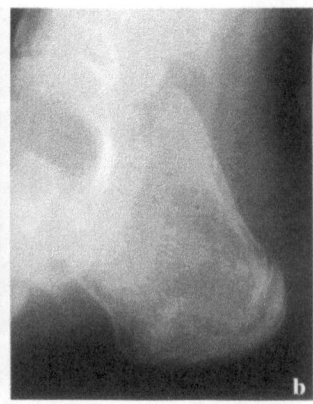

Fig. 5. a Coronal MR (STIR sequence, TR 3000, TE30 and T1 150) image of both lower legs obtained from a child with left tibial allograft shows stress changes (increased signal intensity) in the right distal tibia and talar dome. **b** Plain X-ray of left calcaneus obtained from a child with right femoral allograft shows stress changes in the posterior aspect of the calcaneus

Fig. 4. Plain X-ray obtained from a child with a right femoral allograft shows bent intramedullary rod within the proximal native tibia. It also shows fracture of the femoral allograft

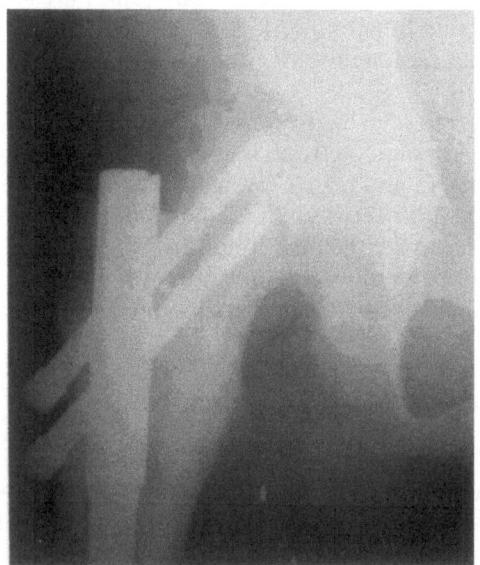

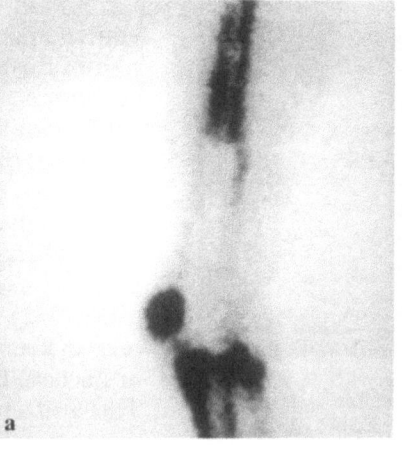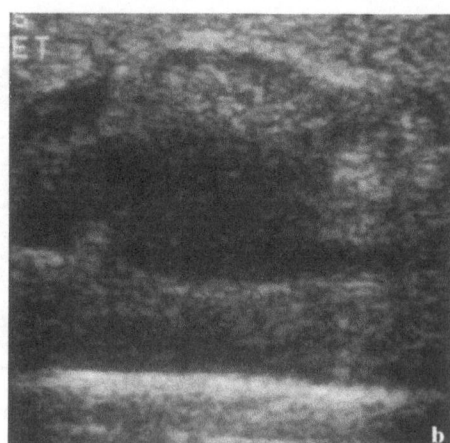

Fig. 7 a, b. Tc^{99m} MDP bone scan and ultrasound obtained from a child with infected femoral endoprosthesis. **a** Lateral view of the bone scan shows no increased activity in the affected area. **b** Subsequent ultrasound shows fluid collection behind the femoral endoprosthesis

Fig. 6. Plain X-ray obtained from a child with a right femoral allograft attached to a native femoral head. It shows degeneration of the femoral head from avascular necrosis

first 3 to 4 years postoperatively [19]. This may relate to the incorporation and revascularization of the grafts and increasing use placed on the grafts by young active patients. Fractures in Van-Nes limbs may relate to the demineralized state of the limb seen postoperatively. Meticulous attention to plain film evaluation is necessary as a fracture line can easily be hidden behind surgical hardware.

Delayed or non-union is defined as lack of union seen more than 1 year following surgery [20] appearing as a radiolucent line at the host-graft junction with lack of cortical bone continuity on all sides (Fig. 3). Adjuvant chemotherapy has been suggested as a cause of delayed union [19]; however, other physiological factors likely play a role with one study reporting that up to half of all delayed unions were seen in patients not receiving chemotherapy [21].

Joint subluxation and hardware failures occur not infrequently and are readily detected by plain radiographs (Figs. 3, 4). Bone demineralization occurs in all affected limbs likely from disuse. It is possible that the adjuvant pre-LSS systemic multi-agent chemotherapy accelerates the demineralization process. Demineralization may lead to insufficiency fractures. Stress-related changes can occur in the contralateral unaffected limbs and be evident on bone scanning or MR imaging most likely secondary to added stress and gait imbalance following treatment (Fig. 5). Another complication detectable later on by plain radiographs is avascular necrosis (Fig. 6).

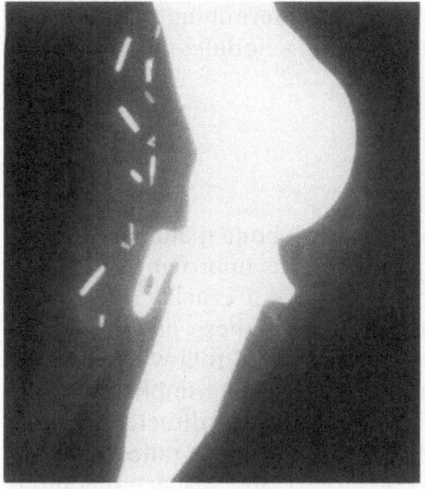
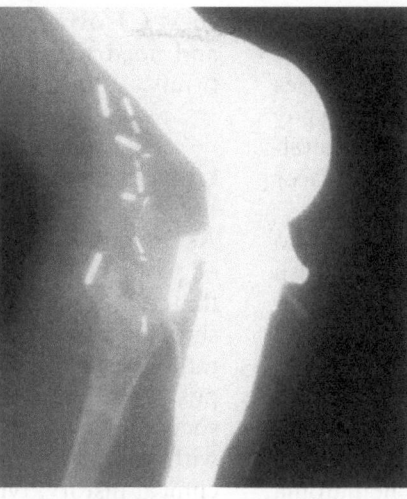

Fig. 8 a, b. Plain X-rays obtained from a child with a massive endoprosthesis who had a local recurrence of the tumor (same child as in Fig. 9) show **a** a radiograph taken prior to the local recurrence, and **b** a recurrence mass in the posterior knee displacing the surgical clips

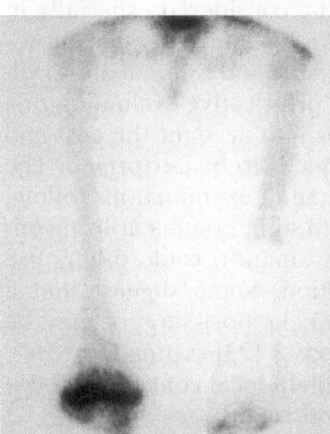
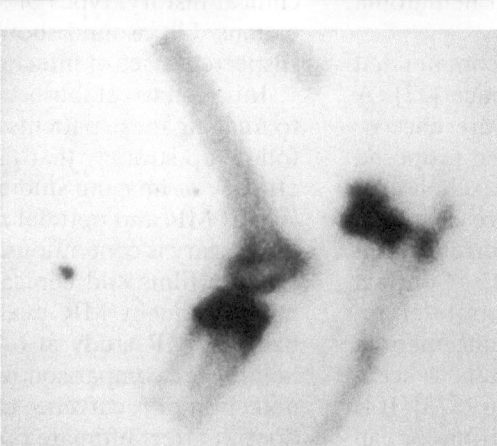

Fig. 9 a, b. Tc^{99m} MDP bone scan obtained from a child with a massive left femoral endoprosthesis who had a local recurrence of the tumor. The local recurrence was obscured by the massive endoprosthesis on the AP view **a**, and was only visible on the lateral view **b**

Leg-length discrepancy is a problem in younger patients with greater growth potential. While a discrepancy of up to 10 cm can be tolerated in the upper extremities, a leg-length discrepancy of more than 2 cm in the lower extremities warrants treatment [20] with early fusion of the contralateral extremity or limb-lengthening procedures.

Although infrequent, imaging of infection following LSS can be a challenge [22]. The traditional modality of bone scan is often suboptimal due to the altered bone uptake at the surgical site where infection most often is seen. Infection may be misinterpreted as postsurgical change by nuclear scan. As fluid or abscess collections are not infrequently associated with infection, ultrasound may be of benefit (Fig. 7).

Tumor Recurrence and Relapse

Before the adoption of chemotherapy almost all patients with malignant bone tumors presented with lung metastases as the first site of metastasis. The use of chemotherapy has altered this relapse pattern with more patients than previously now presenting with a local recurrence or distant bone metastasis before lung metastases develop.

The local recurrence rate for osteosarcoma treated with systemic multi-agent chemotherapy and surgery ranges from 4-11% to 19% with history of pathologic fracture [23]. For Ewing's sarcoma the recurrence rate with surgery is between 4-17% but can be as high as 36% if primary treatment is radiotherapy with or without systemic multi-agent chemotherapy [23]. For malignant sarcomas following LSS the site of recurrence tends to be in the soft tissues as the native bone has been excised but recurrence may also occur at the bone prosthesis interface [23]. Plain films tend to reveal recurrence only by virtue of their mass effect with contour alterations, clip displacement or involvement of adjacent bone (Fig. 8) [23].

Bone scintigraphy has been effective in detecting both relapse and metastatic bone disease with 50% of relapses being detected before clinically evident possibly at a time when alternative therapy may be offered. Increased activity is nonspecific and can be seen with altered weight-bearing, aseptic loosening, infection or local recurrence. Misinterpretation of this activity may lead to further unnecessary investigations with high cost and radiation load. Indeed one study by Kaste et al. [24] showed that only 44% of the patients developed normal pattern of activity after LSS. These authors suggested that the baseline post-LSS scintigraphic appearance must be defined so that one can accurately interpret postoperative bone scans of patients with LSS. In cases with massive metallic prosthesis, radiologists should pay careful attention to the use of lateral views as the metallic prosthesis may easily obscure abnormal radiotracer uptake (Fig. 9).

Ultrasound can be used in routine follow-up to demonstrate recurrent soft tissue tumor and distinguish cystic from solid lesions [23]. It can also be used for tumor biopsy [23].

On CT recurrent tumor may demonstrate altered soft tissue density, tumor mineralization or bone destruction. Metallic artifacts can be problematic especially adjacent to joints [23]. CT cannot reliably differentiate recurrent tumor from granulation tissue and hematoma [23].

Magnetic resonance is currently the recommended modality for evaluating for tumor recurrence [23]. A strategy for evaluation dependent on the presence or absence of high T2-weighted signal has been proposed [23]. The absence of high signal generally excludes tumor recurrence [23]. However, the presence of a high signal mass doesn't necessarily indicate recurrence as it can be seen in hematomas and seromas [23]. Contrast enhanced T1-weighted images will demonstrate either no enhancement or minimal peripheral enhancement in seromas [23]. If more extensive enhancement is seen, then biopsy and tumor re-staging is necessary [23]. It is important to note that seroma and recurrent tumor can occur at the same time.

High signal on T2-weighted images can be seen with infection and abscess [23]. Enhancement per se does not indicate tumor as it can be seen with inflammation shortly after surgery, soft tissue infection and radiation-induced pseudomass [23]. Employing a dynamic sequence and measuring the rate of enhancement may help. Recurrent tumor enhances early (within 2 min) while granulation tissue typically enhances more slowly [23]. Rapid enhancement may also be seen in inflamed tissues whether recently postoperative or infected where the enhancement tends to be more diffuse and less masslike [23]. It is important to recognize that postoperative changes occur in adjacent soft tissue including muscles used to cover residual bone. If a muscle is denervated as a result of surgery it may appear enlarged and edematous and subsequently show fatty atrophy [23].

Distant Metastases

For distant metastases to the lungs CT of the chest is most helpful providing early detection of malignant lung nodules. However, CT of the chest detects not only malignant lung nodules before chest X-ray, but also small benign nodules which may precipitate additional follow-up studies or even thoracotomy. The added value of chest CT over chest X-ray in determining the presence and need for resection of lung nodules has not been firmly established.

Conclusions

As the outlook for patients with bone malignancy treated with chemotherapy and LSS is improving, it is clear that radiographic imaging plays a crucial role in the short and long-term follow-up of these patients. Plain radiographs remain the mainstay of follow up imaging post-LSS demonstrating most of the complications associated with LSS. The need for more directed imaging with scintigraphy, MR or CT should be tailored to the clinical history, types of surgery and suspected complications. Ultrasound should be considered especially in suspected cases of infection or local tumor recurrence

It is vital to establish a reliable and rational approach to imaging these patients. A prospective evaluation of a follow-up strategy that takes into account the cost and efficacy of imaging studies needs to be performed. The role of MR and optimal timing of examinations following surgery is contentious with some centers utilizing only plain films and clinical evaluation while others use more frequent MR evaluation. Some suggest that a baseline MR study at 6-8 weeks post-surgery may be helpful for comparison purposes [23] stating that early detection of recurrence can help local control even if it doesn't affect ultimate prognosis [23].

References

1. Dahlin DC, Unni KK (1986) Bone tumors. General aspects and data on 8 542 cases. Charles C Thomas, Springfield
2. Huvos AG (1991) Bone tumor: diagnosis, treatment and prognosis. WB Saunders, Philadelphia, pp 85-155
3. Fletcher BD (1991) Response of osteosarcoma and Ewing sarcoma to chemotherapy: imaging evaluation. AJR 157: 825-833
4. Gitalis S (1991) Limb salvage for appendicular tumors. Curr Opin Orthop 2: 811-816
5. Korholz D, Verheyen J, et al. (1998) Evaluation of follow-up investigations in osteosarcoma patients: suggestions for an effective follow-up program. Med Pediatr Oncol 30: 52-58
6. van der Woude HJ, Bloem JL, Hogerdoom PC (1998) Preoperative evaluation and monitoring chemotherapy in patients with high-grade osteogenic and Ewing's sarcoma: review of current imaging modalities. Skeletal Radiol 27: 57-71
7. Petrilli AS, Gentil FC, Epelman S, et al. (1991) Increased survival, limb preservation, and prognostic factors for osteosarcoma. Cancer 68: 733-737
8. Pastorino U, Gasparini M, Tavecchio L, et al. (1994) The contribution of salvage surgery to the management of childhood osteosarcoma. J Clin Oncol 9: 1357-1362
9. McDonald DJ (1994) Limb-salvage surgery for treatment of sarcomas of the extremities. AJR 163: 509-513
10. Simon MA, Aschliman MA, Thomas N, Mankin HJ (1986) Limb-salvage treatment versus amputation for osteosarco-

ma of the distal end of the femur. J Bone Joint Surg Am 69: 1331-1337

11. Fletcher BD (1997) Imaging pediatric bone sarcomas. Diagnosis and treatment-related issues. Radiol Clin North Am 35: 1477-1494

12. van der Woude HJ, Bloem JL, Van Uostayen JA (1995) Treatment of high-grade bone sarcomas with neoadjuvant chemotherapy: the utility of sequential color Doppler sonography in predicting histopathologic response. Am J Roentgenol 165: 125-133

13. Kinoshita T, Tatezaki S, Matsuzoki O, et al. (1995) Ultrasonographic monitoring of the effects of preoperative chemotherapy in osteosarcoma and Ewing's sarcoma. Int Orthop 19: 312-314

14. van der Woude HJ, Bloem JL, Schipper J (1994) Changes in tumor perfusion induced by chemotherapy in bone sarcomas: color Doppler flow imaging compared with contrast-enhanced MR imaging and three-phase bone scintigraphy. Radiology 191: 421-431

15. Exner GU, Von Hochstetter AR, Augustiny N, Von Schulthess G (1990) Magnetic resonance imaging in malignant bone tumour. Int Orthop 14: 49-56

16. Cara JA, Canadell J (1994) Limb salvage for malignant bone tumors in young children. J Ped Orthop 14: 112-118

17. Kohler R, Lorge F, Brunat-Mentigny M, Noyer D, Patricot L (1990) Massive bone allografts in children. Int Orthop 14: 249-253

18. Ward WG, Yang R-S, Eckardt JJ (1996) Endoprosthetic bone reconstruction following malignant tumor resection in skeletally immature patients. Orthop Clinic North Am 27(3): 493-502

19. Ortiz-Cruz E, Gebhardt MC, Jennings LC, Springfield DS, Mankin HJ (1997) The results of transplantation of intercalary allografts after resection of tumors. J Bone Joint Surg 79: A97-A106

20. Alman BA, De Bari A, Krajbich JI (1995) Massive allografts in the treatment of osteosarcoma and Ewing sarcoma in children and adolescents. J Bone Joint Surg 77: 54-64

21. Quill G, Gitelis, S, Morton T, Piasecki P (1990) Complications associated with limb salvage for extremity sarcomas and their management. Clin Orthop 260: 242-250

22. Lord CF, Gebhardt MC, Tomford WW, Mankin HJ (1988) Infection in bone allografts. J Bone Joint Surg 70: A369-A376

23. Davies AM, Vanel D (1998) Follow-up of musculoskeletal tumors. I. Local recurrence. Eur Radiol 8: 791-799

24. Kaste SC, Rao BN, Meyer WM, Lynch M (1996) Limb-sparing procedures: postoperative planar bone scan appearance. Pediatr Radiol 26: 750-753

Imaging of Arthritis in Children

K. Rosendahl

Department of Paediatric Radiology, University Hospital of Bergen, Bergen, Norway

Definitions

Arthritis (Greek arthron, joint, + -itis, inflammation): inflammation of one (monarthritis) or more (poly-) joints. Juvenile rheumatoid arthritis (JRA): a systemic connective tissue disorder, which may affect any synovial joint of the body. The term is commonly used in the United States. Juvenile chronic arthritis (JCA): in addition to JRA, this term includes other paediatric connective tissue disorders, such as juvenile ankylosing spondylitis and psoreatic arthritis. The term is commonly used in the United kingdom and other parts of the world. Criteria for the diagnosis of JCA are onset under 16 years and duration of minimum 3 months

Aetiology

Arthritis may result from or be associated with a number of conditions including connective tissue diseases; trauma; congenital disorders; inflammatory diseases;

Table 1. Diseases that may cause arthritis in children (the list is not complete)

Connective tissue diseases
  Juvenile rheumatoid arthritis
  Acute rheumatic fever
  Juvenile spondyloarthropathy
  Psoriasis
  Reiter's syndrome
Trauma
Congenital disorders
Inflammatory diseases
  Transient synovitis
  Pyogenic arthritis
  Osteomyelitis
  Tuberculosis
  Fungal infections
  Pigmented villonodular synovitis
Haematological
Neoplastic diseases
  Leukaemia
  Neuroblastoma
  Osteoid osteoma

haematological; and neoplastic diseases (Table 1). In this presentation I will focus on JRA, but also comment on some of the other diseases that can be associated with joint symptoms in children.

Juvenile Rheumatoid Arthritis (JRA)

The reported prevalence of JRA varies between 20 and 70 per 100 000 children. The disease may have a pauciarticular (affection of four or less joints), monarticular, polyarticular (affection of five or more joints) or systemic onset.

About 65% of children with JRA present with pauciarticular affection, with up to 35% being monarticular (usually the knee). The majority of these children are below 5 years of age, with an equal sex incidence, and present with transitory pain, swelling and stiffness of joint(s). Up to 40% of these children develop polyarticular disease.

Children with a polyarticular onset JRA present at any time in childhood, and are classified as being rheumatoid factor positive or negative. The seropositive patients are more often female with a clinical onset after 10 years of age, and with affection of the ulnar styli, wrists and metacarpophalangeal joints. Erosive changes are seen early. The seronegative patients have an adult form of the disease, with affection of the knees, wrists, ankles, tarsi and cervical spine. Involvement of the proximal and distal interphalyngeal joints and of the flexor tendons of the hand may also be seen. Affection of the hip and elbow occur late.

The systemic onset JRA (Still's disease) often presents with intermittent fever and enlargement of the spleen and lymph nodes. Joint affection may occur later. Approximately 50% of the patients are in remission after 5 years' duration.

Imaging: Role and Modalities

The role of imaging in JRA is first to diagnose, second to evaluate the activity of the disease and third to monitor the effect of therapy.

Plain radiographs of the affected joint(s) are the initial examination, and may rule out other causes of joint affection. Moreover, it may visualise early changes of JRA such as soft-tissue swelling, periarticular osteoporosis, accelerated maturation of the epiphysis and periostitis. Ultrasound allows assessment of joint effusions, and may also differentiate between fluid and a thickened synovia in some joints, i.e. the knee and the hip. Moreover, ultrasound may facilitate aspiration if indicated, especially in monarthritis, where other diseases such as purulent arthritis have to be ruled out. Magnetic resonance imaging (MRI) is superior to other modalities in showing subtle cartilage and soft-tissue changes in the early stages of the disease, when radiographs are still normal. Today, however, the majority of children up to 4-5 years of age need sedation which limits the use of the method. Computed tomography (CT) may be of value in visualising the axial skeleton and the sacroiliac joints. Bone scintigraphy may be useful in evaluating the activity of the disease, however, the method is flawed with both false positives and false negatives.

Imaging: Findings

Radiological changes depend on the age of the patient, the duration and localisation of the symptoms and whether or not treatment has been given. The initial finding is often soft tissue swelling, followed by periarticular osteoporosis, growth disturbances and periostitis. Erosive changes of cartilage and bone, bone fusion and alignment deformities appear later. Necrosis of the femoral head and compression fractures of the axial skeleton may be related to steroid therapy and immobilisation.

Soft Tissue Swelling. Following the first weeks of disease, swelling of the periarticular soft-tissues is visible. The swelling results from periarticular oedema, synovial proliferation and accumulation of joint fluid, and is seen as periarticular, fusiform densities on plain radiographs (Fig. 1). The changes may be uni-or bilateral, and if subtle, require a meticulous radiographic technique.

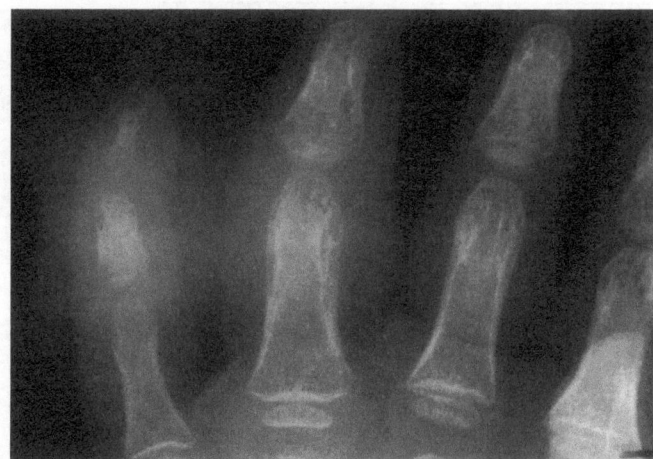

Fig. 1. Fusiform soft-tissue swelling around the fourth proximal interphalangeal joint in a 3-year-old girl with a pauciarticular JRA. There is also periostitis in the fourth proximal phalanx

Joint Effusion/Synovial Thickening. Ultrasound is the method of choice in detection of joint effusions, especially in the hip and in the knee. With high frequency linear probes (12-15 MHz), it is possible to measure the thickness of the synovia and to roughly estimate the amount of fluid (Fig. 2). Popliteal cysts (Baker's cysts), with their characteristic projection towards the tendon of the gastrocnemius muscle, may be seen in up to 40% of the patients. Ultrasound may also guide the injection of steroids into joints. MRI if available, is superior to any other modality in showing both effusion and synovitis (Fig. 3). Synovitis is seen as areas of low signal intensity (dark) on T1-weighted images. As opposed to fluid, a hypervascular synovia enhances after administration of intravenous contrast. MRI also has the advantage of visualising cartilage.

Growth Disturbances. In younger children, growth disturbances secondary to the hyperaemia of the inflammatory process may be seen after a few months. Accelerated maturation of the local epiphyseal ossification centres, round bones and sesamoids, together with widening and elongation of the bone ends near the

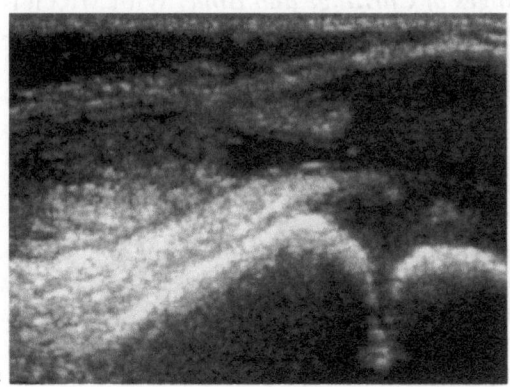
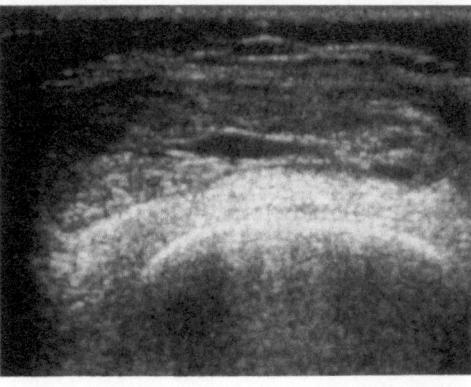

Fig. 2 a, b. Sagittal and axial sections through the knee joint and suprapatellar bursa, showing a thickened synovia and a small amount of fluid on ultrasound

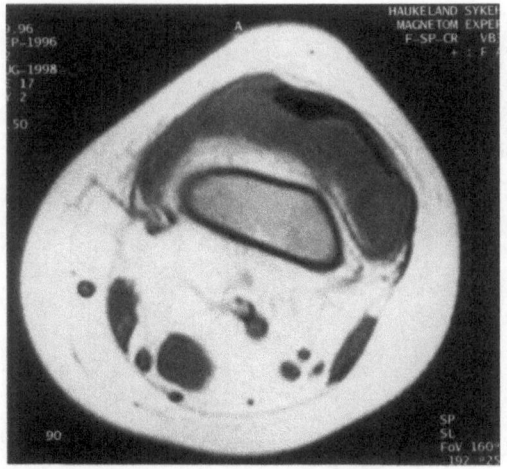 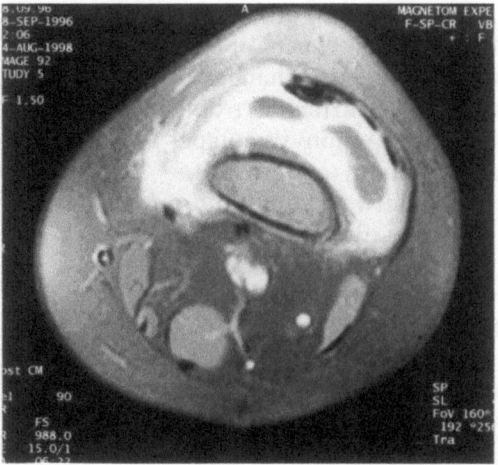

Fig. 3. a T1 weighted, axial sections through the knee joint, showing a distended bursa suprapatellaris with a low signal. **b** After administration of intravenous contrast, the thickened and hyperaemic synovia enhances (white), while the fluid does not

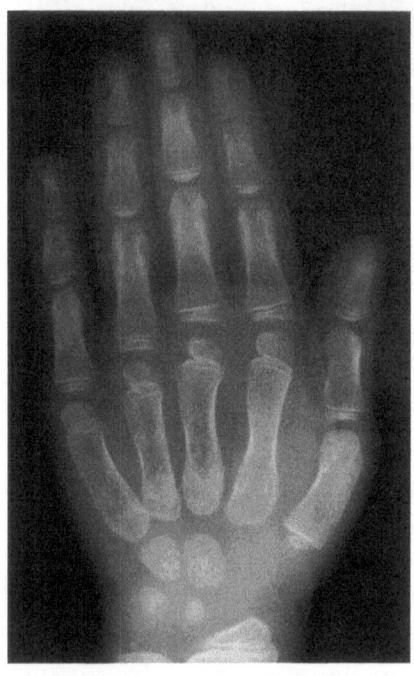

Fig. 4. Angulation of the metacarpal epiphysis and osteopenia in a 4-year-old girl with a polyarticular JRA

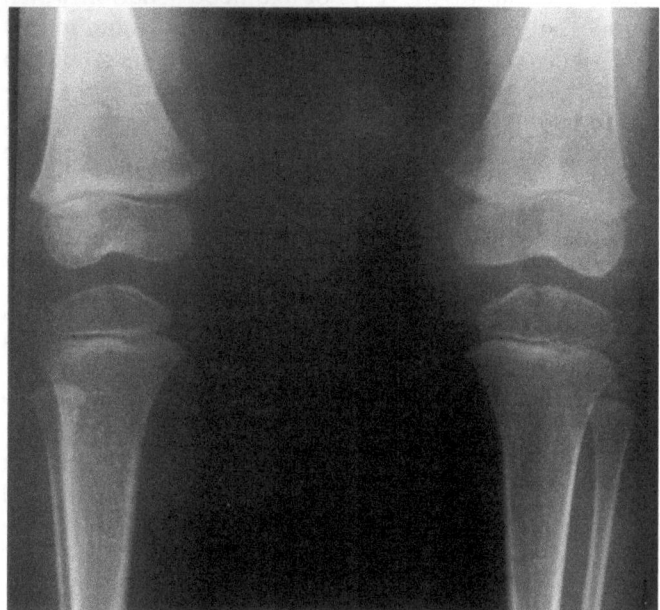

Fig. 5. Overgrowth of the left distal femoral epiphysis

joints may be seen (Fig. 4). A bulbous appearance of the distal portion of the proximal phalanxes is a typical finding in JRA. In the knee the distal femoral epiphysis or the patella may be enlarged (Fig. 5). In cases of unilateral affection, radiographs of both knees are mandatory to detect subtle differences in size. Hyperaemia may eventually result in premature closure of growth plates (short metacarpals/tarsals and small mandible).

Periostitis. Periostitis is seen on plain radiographs and is an unspecific finding in JRA (Fig. 1). It may be diaphyseal when associated with synovitis of adjacent flexor tendons sheath, or metaphyseal when related to affected joints.

Demineralisation. Occurs initially around the affected joints with loss of subarticular trabeculae and thinning of the articular cortices (endosteal resorption). Subse-

quently a more general bone loss may be seen. The degree of bone loss may be evaluated on plain radiographs, and dual X-ray absorptiometry is seldom necessary.

Erosive Changes of Cartilage and Bone. With MRI it is possible to visualise cartilaginous structures in various planes. Normal cartilage has an intermediate signal (grey) on T1-weighted images, and a high signal (white) on gradient echo sequences. On both sequences, the thin articular cartilage appears somewhat brighter than the underlying growth cartilage. On plain radiographs, the thickness of the cartilage may be determined indirectly by measuring the height of the joint space. Because the cartilage around the epiphysis is relatively thick in children, bone erosions often appear relatively late. In children with seropositive JRA, however, bone erosions appear earlier.

Other Signs. Affection of the cervical spine may be asymptomatic, and is rarely seen in patients with pauciarticular affection. When present, it involves C1/C2 with pannus formation and subluxation. Lateral radiographs with flexion and extension may detect a pathological movement between the anterior arch of C1 and the dens. After about 5 years of disease, erosion and fusion of the apophyseal joints may also be seen, predominantly at C2/C3. Involvement of the temporomandibular joints, with erosions and changes at the epiphysis of the condyle, may result in growth disturbances (hypoplasia) of the mandible. It is more common in children with polyarticular than pauciarticular disease.

Spondylarthritis

Ankylosing spondylitis, psoreatic arthritis, Reiter´s disease and enteropathic arthritis represent a subgroup of arthritis in children.

Juvenile ankylosing spondylitis occurs in about 20% of patients with juvenile chronic arthritis, most often in those who are suffering from the pauciarticular disease. About 10% of patients with ankylosing spondylitis are diagnosed before 15 years of age. They are predominantly males older than 10 years of age, of whom 25% are HLA-B27 positive. Changes in the sacroiliac joints may develop before onset of local symptoms, and may be difficult to evaluate on plain films, CT or MRI may be of help.

Trauma

Trauma is a common cause of monarthritis. Sports injuries as well as (non-)accidental injuries must be kept in mind when diagnosing children with a painful joint. If meniscus or ligament ruptures are clinically suspected, MRI may give valuable information.

Inflammatory Disease

Transient synovitis of the hip is an inflammatory condition of unknown origin, and affects children between 2 and 10 years of age. The condition is self-limiting, and most patients recover after 1 to 3 weeks without any sequels. The reported incidence of Legg-Calvé-Perthes as a complication to the disorder is 1-2%. Boys are more frequently affected than are girls. These children often present with acute onset local pain and limp. Anamnes-tic data, clinical examination and laboratory findings may commonly rule out trauma and pyogenic infection. Ultrasound should be the method of choice to show the joint effusion. If still in doubt, plain films and joint aspiration should be performed. Treatment and follow-up on an outpatient basis has gained more and more acceptance.

Purulent arthritis is seen more frequently in the paediatric population than in adults. In the neonate, extension of a metaphyseal focus of osteomyelitis is a common route of infection, while haematogenous spread is more likely in older children. At all ages, there is a great diversity of infecting bacteria, but *Staphylococci* and *Haemophilus influenza* e predominate in infants under 2 years of age. The hip is most frequently affected, especially in neonates. Diagnosis is based on joint aspiration, ultrasound guided if possible. In addition to the effusion, ultrasound may show thickening of the capsular and pericapsular tissues and blurring of the soft tissues around the joint. The associated changes may be detected with MRI or bone scintigraphy at an earlier stage than with ordinary plain films.

Neoplasms

Leukaemia is an important differential diagnosis in children who present with joint symptoms, and must be suspected when lucent metaphyseal bands, often multiple, are seen on plain films. Osteoid osteoma may, when localised in an intracapsular portion of the bone, cause synovial irritation and effusion.

References

1. Poznanski AK (1992) Radiologic approach to joint disease in children. In: Resnick D, Petterson H (eds) Skeletal radiology. Merit Communications, London, pp 455-481
2. Kaye JK (1992) Septic arthritis. In: Resnick D, Petterson H (eds.) Skeletal radiology. Merit Communications, London, pp 498-511
3. Renton P (eds) Diseases of joints. In: Carty H, Brunelle F (eds) Imaging children. Churchill Livingston, New York, pp 1260-1281
4. Caffey (1993) Diseases of the joints. In: Silverman FN, Kuhn JP (eds) Caffey's pediatric X-ray diagnosis. Mosby, St. Louis, pp 1950-1960
5. Cellerini M, Salti S, Trapani S, D'Elia G, Falcini F, Villari N (1999) Correlation between clinical and ultrasound assessment of the knee in children with mono-articular or pauci-articular juvenile rheumatoid arthritis. Pediatric Radiology 29: 117-123

Benign Tumors of the Epi/metaphysis

D. Jaramillo

Department of Radiology, Children's Hospital and Harvard Medical School, Boston, USA

Introduction

The imaging evaluation of neoplastic lesions of the appendicular skeleton has two main goals. The first is to determine whether the lesion warrants doing nothing at all, follow-up, or biopsy. The second, mostly relevant to malignant bone tumors, is to provide detailed information about the lesion's extent and biological activity in order to guide therapy. Arriving at a specific diagnosis is an interesting exercise, but it is not the main objective of the radiologic evaluation. This discussion is in two sections, one on evaluation of benign lesions, and the other on imaging of skeletal malignancies. The discussion concentrates on practical issues relevant to the radiologist's role in the management of these lesions. More comprehensive discussions regarding the imaging characteristics of each individual lesion, and illustrations of such lesions are beyond the scope of this discussion. The reader is referred to the standard texts for more detailed coverage of these topics.

Benign Lesions of the Pediatric Skeleton

The study of benign tumors affecting the bones of the extremities is important for various reasons. First, we must distinguish normal variants and non-neoplastic abnormalities from tumors. Second, we must distinguish benign from malignant neoplasms. Third, we must identify those lesions that are significant because of the signs and symptoms related to them including pain and inflammation. Finally, we must be able to identify lesions at risk of complications such as pathologic fracture, osteoarthritis, growth disturbance or malignant transformation. Each one of these scenarios will be discussed.

Normal Variants compared with Tumor

In the epiphysis, normal irregularities of ossification can resemble bone destruction. The proximal femoral epiphysis and the distal femoral epiphysis are common sites of irregular bony contour on radiographs. The medial distal femoral condyle during early childhood and later, the posterior lateral distal femoral condyle, can appear fragmented [1]. The greater tuberosity of the humerus can produce a lucency which is often mistaken for bone destruction. In the round bones, the central portion of the calcaneus is often lucent and can also resemble a cyst (calcaneal pseudocyst) [2].

Areas of physeal widening secondary to a variety of metaphyseal insults can also be mistaken for neoplasms, particularly on magnetic resonance (MR) imaging [3]. The normal physis on cross-sectional axial images can appear as an area of marrow irregularity with areas of sclerosis mixed with areas of lucency on computed tomography (CT), and low T1 signal intensity and high T2 signal intensity on MR images [4]. Normal synchondroses can appear as slightly expansile lucencies on radiographs, particularly in the ischiopubic region [5].

In the metaphysis and metadiaphysis, the insertion of muscles and ligaments can produce cortical irregularities [6]. When imaged *en face*, radiographs show a rounded area of lucency. When seen tangentially, the radiographs show irregularity or discontinuity of the cortex. On coronal or sagittal MR images, the cortical irregularities are seen as hypointense on T1, hyperintense on T2 and markedly enhancing after gadolinium administration [7]. Metaphyseal hematopoietic marrow can resemble metastatic disease or primary neoplasm on MR images. Hematopoietic marrow, however, contains 40% fat, and is therefore of higher signal intensity than neoplasms on T1-weighted images [8]. On conventional spin echo T2-weighted images, hematopoietic marrow is of intermediate signal intensity, but on fast spin echo T2-weighted or short tau inversion recovery (STIR) images it can have higher signal intensity and closely resemble pathology.

In the diaphysis of the femur, humerus and tibia of infants, physiologic periosteal new bone formation can be seen as symmetric lines adjacent and parallel to the cortex of the bones [9]. Nutrient foramina are very prominent in newborns and young infants, and are seen as well-rounded diaphyseal lucencies on radiographs, and are hyperintense on T_2-weighted MR imaging.

Non-neoplastic Abnormalities compared with Tumor

In the epiphysis, epiphyseal osteomyelitis and tuberculosis can produce lucencies with relatively few symptoms. These are difficult to distinguish from epiphyseal tumors such as chondroblastomas or histiocytosis. All of these epiphyseal lesions grow slowly and have well-defined margins on radiographs. Furthermore, all induce inflammation of adjacent tissues seen as perilesional edema on MR images [10]. Radiographic calcification of an epiphyseal lesion suggests chondroblastoma, and central necrosis on MR images suggests osteomyelitis.

Avulsive injuries of the apophyses often resemble neoplasms. In the pelvis of older children and adolescents, repeated avulsions of the apophyses at the insertion of large muscle groups are often associated with irregularity of the bony contour and with marked bone proliferation [11].

Stress fractures, particularly in young adolescents who may not be forthcoming with a history of increased activity, are often confused with neoplasms [12]. Radiographically both can produce cortical discontinuity and periosteal reaction. Short-term follow up will clearly show rapid changes in the periosteum in fractures; the periosteum will become radiographically more solid and continuous, and the fracture line may become evident. On MR images, stress injuries often reveal an elevated periosteum without a real soft tissue mass; the disruption of the periosteum by the injury is frequently apparent.

In the soft tissues, peripheral calcification of a mass suggests myositis ossificans rather than tumor. On radiographs and particularly on CT, myositis ossificans has a better defined outer border than an inner border (peripheral margination). In contrast, soft tissue neoplastic calcification or bone formation is densest in the center. Myositis ossificans on MR images can resemble a malignant tumor because it has a soft tissue mass and because the ossification is less apparent than on CT images [13].

Benign compared with Malignant Lesions

On radiographs, it is difficult to differentiate with certainty between benign and malignant lesions. Ultimately most neoplasms are examined histologically. There are, however, certain imaging characteristics that can help (Table 1). Most epiphyseal lesions are benign. Epiphyseal neoplasms in children include osteochondromas (in dysplasia epiphysialis hemimelica or Trevor's disease), chondroblastomas, and histiocytosis. Well-defined margins on radiographs and CT scans indicate slow growth and are usually associated with benign diseases. In contrast, on MR images, ill-defined margins indicate perilesional edema, often benign. Lesions with well-defined margins on MR images are usually malignant [14]. The converse is not true; many osteogenic sarcomas can also have extensive peripheral edema. Solid periosteal reaction indicates a benign process. On MR images, an abnormality that is entirely cystic can be considered benign, whereas a mass that breaks through the cortex or periosteum can be considered malignant.

Pain and Inflammation

Three benign neoplasms present primarily with pain and inflammation: osteoid osteoma, chondroblastoma, and localized forms of histiocytosis [14]. Osteoid osteomas

Table 1. Bone tumors in children according to location (modified from [4])

Location	Central	Eccentric	Cortical	Periosteal	Soft Tissue
Epiphysis	Chondroblastoma *Histiocytosis*		Trevor disease		
Metaphysis	Enchondroma UBC Osteosarcoma *Ewing*	ABC Osteosarcoma *Ewing*	Osteo-chondroma chondroma Osteosarcoma *Ewing*	Periosteal chondroma Osteosarcoma *Ewing*	Osteosarcoma *Ewing*
Meta-Diaphysis	Fibrous dysplasia	Chondromyxoid fibroma	Non-ossifying fibroma		Myositis ossificans
Diaphysis	*Histiocytosis* *Ewing*		Osteoid osteoma Osteofibrous dysplasia Adamantinoma		Neuro-fibromatosis Rhabdomyosarcoma

PVNS, pigmented villonodular synovitis; *UBC*, unicameral bone cyst; *ABC*, aneurysmal bone cyst
underlined lesions are malignant; italicized lesions are round cell tumors

are spontaneously healing lesions; the goal of therapy is to alleviate pain, and sometimes oral analgesics can suffice. Eosinophilic granuloma, the solitary form of Langerhans cell hystiocytosis, can be managed with observation or steroid injection [15]. Chondroblastomas, on the other hand, tend to grow and invade the joint and must be resected. All of these lesions are lucent radiographically but they can incite abundant reactive bone formation. Chondroblastomas and intra-articular osteoid osteomas produce irritation of the joint and they can produce abundant synovial inflammation. All of these lesions produce extensive marrow and soft tissue abnormality on MR images, due to the prominent perilesional disease. The lesions are highly vascular and enhance with gadolinium. In osteoid osteomas [16] and some chondroblastomas [17], the perilesional reaction obscures the lesion. Misdiagnosis with MR imaging is frequent, particularly if high resolution images are not obtained. CT scanning is the preferred cross-sectional technique for evaluation of osteoid osteomas. The nidus of the osteoid osteoma, highly vascular and osteogenic, has intense radiotracer uptake on bone scintigraphy.

Interventional radiologists have been active in the therapy of osteoid osteomas. Under CT guidance, the nidus is located, and destroyed, either mechanically, or with thermal ablation [18].

Holes in the Bone and Pathologic Fractures

Various benign pathologies produce well-defined bony lucencies, which although clearly benign, are significant because of the risk of pathologic fracture. This most common entity is the unicameral bone cyst (UBC). This arises centrally in the periphyseal metaphysis of the proximal humerus or proximal femur. It disturbs metaphyseal modeling but seldom extends beyond the perimeter of the physis. It rarely crosses the physis [19]; as it becomes quiescent, the physis migrates away from it, and its location becomes more diaphyseal. Unicameral bone cysts often present with pathological fractures and a fragment of bone within the cystic cavity (fallen fragment sign) [20]. On gadolinium enhanced MR images, the lesion is entirely cystic; after a fracture, however, the granulation tissue within the cyst can resemble a mass. Few fluid-fluid levels can also be seen in a unicameral bone cyst after trauma [21].

Aneurysmal bone cysts are usually expansile and eccentric and they can be found almost anywhere in the skeleton [22]. Large lesions can appear to violate the cortex radiographically, but on CT and MR images the lesions have a well-defined rim. On MR images, the lesions are multiloculated, with fluid-fluid levels indicating the presence of blood-filled spaces [23]. A lesion with many fluid-fluid levels but no soft tissue mass is almost certainly an aneurysmal bone cyst. On the other hand, if a soft tissue mass accompanies the fluid-fluid

levels, the abnormality may represent a malignancy such as a telangiectatic osteogenic sarcoma [24].

A non-ossifying fibroma has a characteristic appearance on radiographs and CT scans. It is a metadiaphyseal lucent lesion with a margin that is more sclerotic on the diaphyseal side; it is cortically based and has serpiginous borders [25]. Another fibrous lesion, fibrous dysplasia, can have characteristic ground glass opacity mixed with cystic areas on radiographs and CT images.

Growth Disturbance and Deformity

Lesions affecting the physis can result in significant growth disturbance. Osteochondromas and enchondromas can stunt growth, particularly when they affect smaller physes such as the ulna and fibula. Osteochondromas arise from the vicinity of the physis and are capped by cartilage that is similar to that of the main physis. In children, the thickness of the cartilaginous cap can exceed 1 cm. Enchondromas in children are seen as tongues of unossified cartilage extending into the metaphysis [26]. The characteristic calcification of cartilaginous lesions (in rings and circles) is not seen in the very young. Cartilaginous lesions show only minimal enhancement on MR images [27].

Bowing in association with neoplasm is more characteristic of fibrous lesions. Bowing of the proximal femur is characteristic of fibrous dysplasia, particularly of the polyostotic variety. In the tibia, osteofibrous dysplasia (Campanacci disease) produces anterior bowing, cystic lesions of the anterior cortex, and ground glass opacity [28].

Malignancy

The risk of malignancy is rare in most benign neoplasms. The highest risk of malignant transformation is that of cartilaginous lesions. In multiple enchondromatosis (Ollier's disease) the combined risk of all the lesions may be as high as 25% [26]. Usually, these patients develop chondrosarcomas after childhood.

Conclusion

In children with imaging studies suggesting a benign skeletal neoplasm, it is crucial to distinguish the abnormality from a normal variant, and from nontumoral pathology such as trauma, infection or infarction. Once it is established that the lesion is indeed benign, it is important to assess the presence and future risk of complications such as pathologic fracture, growth arrest, deformity or malignant transformation, which are the main reasons to undergo treatment.

References

1. Caffey J, Madell SH, Royer C, Morales P (1958) Ossification of the distal femoral epiphysis. JBJS 40: A647-A654
2. Keats T, Harrison RB (1979) The calcaneal nutrient foramen: a useful sign in the differentiation of true from simulated cysts. Skeletal Radiol 3: 239-240
3. Laor T, Hartman AL, Jaramillo D (1997) Local physeal widening on MR imaging: an incidental finding suggesting prior metaphyseal insult. Pediatr Radiol 27: 654-662
4. Laor T, Jaramillo D, Oestreich AE (1998) Musculoskeletal system. In: Kirks DR, Griscom NT (eds) Practical pediatric imaging: diagnostic radiology of infants and children, 3rd edn. Lippincott-Raven, Philadelphia, pp. 327-510
5. Caffey J, Ross SE (1956) The Ischiopubic synchondrosis in healthy children: some normal roentgenologic findings. AJR 76: 488-494
6. Keats T, Joyce J (1984) Metaphyseal cortical irregularities in children: a new perspective on a multifocal growth variant. Skeletal Radiol 12: 112-118
7. Yamazaki T, Maruoka S, Takahashi S, et al. (1995) MR findings of avulsive cortical irregularities of the distal femur. Skeletal Radiol 24: 43-46
8. Fletcher BD, Wall JE, Hanna SL (1993) Effect of hematopoietic growth factors on MR images of bone marrow in children undergoing chemotherapy. Radiology 189: 745-751
9. Shopfner C (1966) Periosteal bone growth in normal infants: a preliminary report. AJR 97: 154-163
10. Ecklund K, Jaramillo D, Buonomo C (1996) Pediatric case of the day. Chondroblastoma. Radiographics 16: 979-982
11. Fernbach S, Wilkinson R (1981) Avulsion injuries of the pelvis and proximal femur. AJR 137: 581-586
12. Daffner R, Pavlov H (1992) Stress fractures: current concepts. AJR 159: 245-252
13. Kransdorf MJ, Meis JM, Jelinek JS (1991) Myositis ossificans: MR appearance with radiologic-pathologic correlation. AJR 157: 1243-1248
14. Jaramillo D, Laor T, Gebhardt MC (1996) Pediatric musculoskeletal neoplasms. Evaluation with MR imaging. Magn Reson Imaging Clin N Am 4: 749-770
15. Meyer JS, Harty MP, Mahboubi S, et al. (1995) Langerhans cell histiocytosis: presentation and evolution of radiologic findings with clinical correlation. Radiographics 15: 1135-1146
16. Assoun J, Richardi G, Railhac JJ, et al. (1994) Osteoid osteoma: MR imaging versus CT. Radiology 191: 217-223
17. Weatherall PT, Maale GE, Mendelsohn DB, Sherry CS, Erdman WE, Pascoe HR (1994) Chondroblastoma: classic and confusing appearance at MR imaging. Radiology 190: 467-474
18. Rosenthal DI, Springfield DS, Gebhardt MC, Rosenbert AE, Mankin HJ (1995) Osteoid osteoma: percutaneous radio-frequency ablation. Radiology 297: 451-454
19. Haims AH, Desai P, Present D, Beltran J (1997) Epiphyseal extension of a unicameral bone cyst. Skeletal Radiol 26: 51-54
20. Reynolds J (1969) The "fallen fragment sign" in the diagnosis of unicameral bone cysts. Radiology 92: 949-953
21. Maas EJ, Craig JG, Swisher PK, Amin MB, Marcus N (1998) Fluid-fluid levels in a simple bone cyst on magnetic resonance imaging. Australas Radiol 42: 267-270
22. Bollini G, Jouve JL, Cottalorda J, Petit P, Panuel M, Jacquemier M (1998) Aneurysmal bone cyst in children: analysis of twenty-seven patients. J Pediatr Orthop 7: 274-285
23. Kransdorf MJ, Sweet DE (1995) Aneurysmal bone cyst: concept, controversy, clinical presentation and imaging. AJR 164: 573-580
24. Tsai JC, Dalinka MK, Fallon MD, Zlatkin MB, Kressel HY (1990) Fluid-fluid level: a nonspecific finding in tumors of bone and soft tissue. Radiology 175: 779-782
25. Ritschl P, Karnel F, Hajek P (1988) Fibrous metaphyseal defects: determination of their origin and natural history using a radiomorphological study. Skeletal Radiol 17: 8-15
26. Brien EW, Mirra JM, Kerr R (1997) Benign and malignant cartilage tumors of bone and joint: their anatomic and theoretical basis with an emphasis on radiology, pathology and clinical biology. I. The intramedullary cartilage tumors. Skeletal Radiol 26: 325-353
27. Geirnaerdt MJ, Bloem JL, Eulderink F, Hogendoorn PC, Taminian AH (1993) Cartilaginous tumors: correlation of gadolinium-enhanced MR imaging and histopathologic findings. Radiology 186: 813-817
28. Campanacci M, Laus M (1981) Osteofibrous dysplasia of the tibia and fibula. J Bone Joint Surg Am 63: 367-375

Bone Marrow Changes in Various Hematological Diseases

G. Benz-Bohm[1], H. Kugel[1], D. Schwamborn[2]

[1] Department of Radiology, University of Cologne, Cologne, Germany
[2] Children's Hospital, University of Cologne, Cologne, Germany

Introduction

Magnetic resonance imaging (MRI) has an excellent spatial and contrast resolution. It is able to separate hematopoietic from fatty marrow and analyse quantitatively the two major marrow components, fat and water. Therefore, it is a highly sensitive technique for evaluation of bone marrow in children.

This chapter discusses the following topics:
- Normal bone marrow
- MR appearance of normal bone marrow
- Bone marrow changes in various hematological diseases and their appearance on MR.

Normal Bone Marrow

The bone marrow is encased in cortical bone and traversed by trabecular bone. Marrow has been classified as either hematopoietic (red) or fatty (yellow). The basic structural unit of the red bone marrow is the capillary-venous sinus that results from progressive bifurcations of the nutrient artery. In red bone marrow, cells with myeloid, erythroid and lymphoid elements add up to nearly 100% with few fat cells at birth. This declines by about 10% per decade throughout life. As the relative amount of myeloid tissue declines, fat cells become apparent. Red marrow is hematopoietically active in the production of all forms of hematopoietic elements, yellow marrow is inactive and is composed predominantly of fat cells. Therefore, the chemical composition of the two types of marrow is different. In adults red marrow contains approximately 40% water, 40% fat, and 20% protein; whereas yellow marrow contains approximately 15% water, 80% fat, and 5% protein. A very important structural difference between these two types of marrow is the vascular supply. The rich sinusoidal system of red marrow is replaced by capillaries, venules and thin-walled veins in fatty marrow [1, 2].

Normal Bone Marrow Conversion

Soon after birth the conversion of hematopoietic to fatty marrow begins in the extremities, especially in the terminal phalanges of the hands and feet, and progresses from peripheral towards the axial skeleton. In the long bones, marrow conversion occurs first in the diaphysis, then in the distal metaphysis and finally in the proximal metaphysis. Histologically, ossifying epiphyses contain some red marrow, especially at birth, but epiphyseal and apophyseal ossification centers can be characterized as yellow marrow, once ossification commences. In adults hematopoietic marrow resides in the skull, vertebral bodies, flat bones, and proximal femoral and humeral metaphyses. Yellow marrow is found in the remainder of the skeleton [2-7].

MR Appearance of Normal Bone Marrow

The larger amount of water in the red marrow originates from the greater number of hematopoietic cells, which contain mostly water. In contrast, fat cells contain mostly fat. The different amounts of fat and water are the main cause of the different appearance of red and yellow marrow on MR images. In ordinary MR images of bone marrow the measured signal originates from both water and fat. Thus, changes of relaxation times of either of these materials contribute to changes in signal intensity. The predominant effect on the images, however, is caused by changes in the relative amounts of fat and water.

Thus, red and yellow marrow can be differentiated with MRI if the right sequences are selected. *Spin-echo sequences* are the standard method used for bone marrow imaging. Because of its increased number of water containing cells, T1 relaxation time is longer in red marrow than in yellow marrow. The T2 relaxation time is variable, depending on the relative amount of water and fat. Therefore, on T1-weighted images, hematopoietic marrow has a signal intensity less than that of fatty marrow or subcutaneous fat, and equal to, or slightly higher than, that of muscle. On T2-weighted images the intensity is slightly less than that of subcutaneous fat but higher than that of muscle. In neonates the signal from red marrow may be slightly less than that from muscle.

Yellow marrow has a relatively short T1 relaxation time and a longer T2 relaxation time than that of the water signal in the red marrow. Therefore, its signal intensity on T1-weighted images is isointense with subcutaneous fat. On T2-weighted images its signal intensity is slightly less than that of subcutaneous fat. Consequently differences in signal intensity between hematopoietic and fatty marrow are best seen on T1-weighted images. They are less obvious or even disappear on T2-weighted images.

The use of turbo spin-echo sequences to speed up T2-weighted imaging enhances fat signal intensity, which further decreases the contrast between fatty marrow and lesions characterized by an increase of free water with a long T2 time. Therefore, *fat suppression techniques* are often used in combination with turbo spin-echo sequences to increase the contrast between normal marrow and pathologic marrow with decreased fat content, as well as between red and yellow marrow.

Two methods of fat suppression are available: a method exploiting the very short T1 relaxation time of fat (short time inversion recovery [STIR] method), and a method based on water and fat signals resonating at different frequencies, a frequency selective fat suppression using saturation or inversion pulses, with various names used by the different manufacturers.

With the STIR method the signal from tissue with the short T1 time typical of fat is nulled. Care must be taken because signals from tissues with short T1 after accumulation of contrast agent may be nulled as well. The remaining signals are usually T2-weighted, with a residual contribution of T1-weighting. Depending on relaxation time differences, this may decrease or increase contrast between different water-containing tissues. Lesions with increased water content can be excellently detected as high intensity areas against surrounding fatty tissue with decreased intensity. However, partly due to the fact that both T1 and T2 times con-tribute to the signal intensity, the specificity is decreased (Fig. 1).

T2-weighted images with pure T2-weighting can be obtained using frequency selective fat suppression. Fatty marrow has low signal intensity, red marrow and marrow lesions have high signal intensity. The major disadvantage of this method is the requirement for a highly uniform magnetic field, which cannot always be accomplished with large fields of view or near surface coils. When using these sequences, one must be careful to exclude image artefacts [2, 6-8].

Before the development of an ossified epiphysis the *physis* is not apparent on T1-weighted MR images. It is represented as a low signal intensity line that separates the ossified epiphysis or apophysis from the bony metaphysis. The *epiphyses* and *apophyses* of the long bones in neonates are hypointense on T1-weighted images (cartilage and some hematopoietic cells). Fatty transformation and consecutively a high signal intensity occurs within 3-4 months after ossification commences [7, 9, 10].

The order of *conversion* has been documented [3-5]. The age at which conversion is seen on MRI is earlier than has been previously reported (Fig. 2) [7, 11, 12].

In the first two decades of life *vertebral marrow* is hematopoietic with a low signal intensity on T1-weighted images. With advancing age, yellow marrow may replace red marrow in a diffuse pattern or in a focal or spotty pattern [13]. In patients older than 10 years the signal intensity of the vertebral marrow should be higher than that of the adjacent intervertebral disk on T1-weighted images. A lower signal intensity suggests replacement by tumor or red marrow hyperplasia [6, 7, 14].

Pelvic marrow is predominantly hematopoietic in the first two decades of life. The "adult pattern", at ages 21-24 years, shows the marrow signal intensity in the anterior ilium and acetabulum approximately equal to that of fat [6, 15].

SIGNAL INTENSITY AND STIR IMAGING	
Very Low	**Intermediate**
Fat	*Muscle*
Cortical bone	Red marrow
Air	Mild infiltration of marrow
Fibrosis (chronic)	
Calcification	**Bright**
Paramagnetic substances	*Musculoskeletal lesions*
Gd-DTPA	*Fluid*
Hemorrhage	*Edema*
	Nodes
	Newborn red marrow
	Infiltrated marrow

Fig. 1. Signal intensity and short time inversion recovery (STIR) imaging [7]. High sensitivity-low specificity

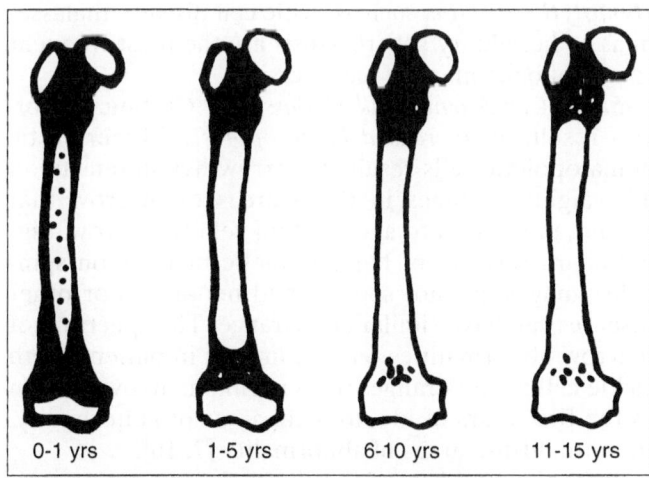

Fig. 2. Femoral marrow conversion on magnetic resonance (MR) images [12]

Bone Marrow Changes in Various Hematological Diseases and their MR-Appearance

In general bone marrow changes in hematological diseases can be classified into [6]:
Bone marrow *reconversion* (*hyperplasia*):
- anemia (hemolytic, megaloblastic);
- Granulocyte-Colony Stimulating Factor-Therapy (G-CSF).

Bone marrow *replacement*:
- leukemia;
- polycythemia vera.

Bone marrow *depletion*:
- aplastic anemia (acquired or congenital);
- aplasia (chemotherapy).

Myelofibrosis:
- radiation therapy and/or chemotherapy.

Bone marrow reconversion

It is the process of repopulation of yellow marrow by hematopoietic cells. The reconversion of fatty to red marrow is started when the hematopoietic capacity of existing red marrow stores is exceeded. The activation of quiescent hematopoietic precursor cells in fatty marrow results in repopulation of fatty marrow by active hematopoietic cells. This generally occurs in a pattern converse to that of physiologic marrow conversion, beginning in the spine and flat bones, progressing to the long bones of the extremities and finally to the hands and feet. In the long bones, reconversion occurs first in the proximal metaphysis of the femur and humerus, then in the distal metaphysis and finally in the diaphysis. Only during severe hematopoietic stress does reconversion occur in the epiphyses and apophyses of the long bones. Marrow reconversion can be uniform or patchy with foci of hematopoietic marrow in fatty marrow [2, 7].

Hemolytic anemias such as sickle cell disease, thalassemias or hereditary spherocytosis are the most frequent causes of bone marrow reconversion.

Sickle Cell Anemia and Thalassemia. Chronic hemolysis results in *increased hematopoiesis*. Hyperplastic hematopoietic cells result in marrow hypointensity on T1-weighted images in those areas of marrow that should, in relation to age, contain yellow marrow. Signal characteristics of hematopoietic marrow on spin-echo images are not specific and neoplastic or other diseases can have similar appearance. The spectrum of marrow abnormalities on MR images in patients with sickle cell anemia ranges from normal marrow pattern in the first years of life, to focal areas of abnormality, to more diffuse areas of abnormality [7, 16].

Infarction and *hemosiderosis* are the two major marrow complications of the hemolytic anemias. *Bone infarcts* in hematopoietic marrow are rare except in patients with sickle cell disease or related hemoglobinopathies. Decreased oxygen delivery as a result of sickle cells results in medullary and periarticular infarction. The long bones are frequently affected. On MRI *acute infarction* shows as focal marrow abnormalities of low-signal intensity on T1-weighted images and high-signal intensity on T2-weighted images. Chronic infarcts are seen as focal lesions with fatty marrow signal intensity centrally and a surrounding hypointense rim on T1-weighted images corresponding to reactive bone [6, 17].

Avascular necrosis of the femoral head occurs in about 15-30% of patients with sickle cell anemia, in all types of epiphyseal marrow. Acute avascular necrosis of the femoral head has a low-signal intensity on T1-weighted images and a high signal intensity on T2-weighted images. The sensitivity of MRI for the detection of femoral head ischemic necrosis is approximately 90% [18-20].

Repeated transfusions result in *hemosiderosis*, in which excess iron is deposited in cells of the reticuloendothelial system. Hemosiderin deposition also occurs in bone marrow. The magnetic susceptibility effects of hemosiderin produce hypointense marrow on T2-weighted images and, particularly in severe iron overload stages, hypointense marrow also in T1-weighted images. The reason for dark marrow even on T1-weighted images, regardless of the fact that T1 time is shortened by the hemosiderin, is that extreme concentrations of paramagnetic iron additionally shorten the T2 relaxation time so much that, even during the short echo times used in T1-weighted imaging, a significant signal loss due to T2 relaxation occurs. Thus, the marrow signal in hemosiderosis is lower than that seen in normal hematopoietic marrow [21, 22].

The MRI appearance of marrow in *thalassemia* is a reflection of the patient's transfusion and chelation therapy. MRI is useful in the evaluation of children with extramedullary hematopoiesis and symptoms of spinal cord compression [23].

Granulocyte-Colony Stimulating Factor-Therapy Effect (G-CSF). Reconversion of fatty marrow to hematopoietic marrow in the metaphysis and diaphysis of long bones can also be seen in children treated with G-CSF. This hematopoietic growth factor stimulates myeloid precursor cells and reduces the myelosuppressive effect of chemotherapy [6, 8].

Bone marrow replacement

It is the infiltration by different neoplastic diseases, e.g. *leukemia*. Leukemia is the most common malignancy in childhood and accounts for more than one third of all malignancies in children. Bone pain is caused by increased intraosseous pressure from proliferation of leukemic cells in the bone marrow. On T1-weighted MR images, leukemic infiltration of the marrow can be dif-

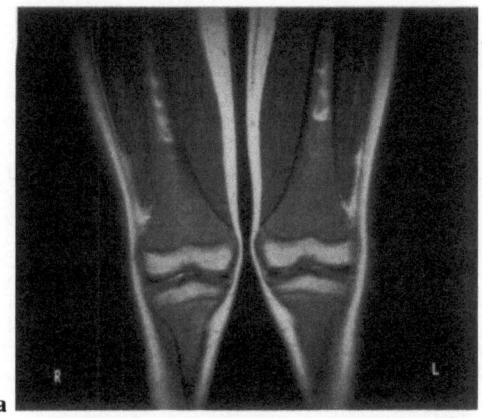

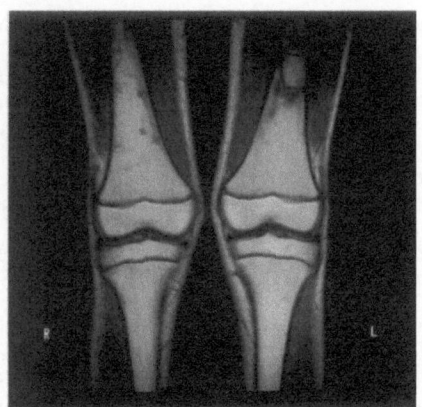

a   b

Fig. 3. a Acute lymphoblastic leukemia (ALL), 5-year-old girl. Diffuse marrow replacement. The epiphyses show normal fatty marrow. Spin-echo sequence, Repetition time 400 ms, Echo time 30 ms. Coronal plane. **b** Acute myeloid leukemia (AML) 10-year-old boy. Focal marrow replacement. Confirmation of the diagnosis by femur biopsy. 62% blasts in the biopsy material. Spin-echo sequence, Repetition time 500 ms, Echo time 30 ms. Coronal plane

fuse or focal marrow replacement by low-to-intermediate signal intensity of leukemic cells (Fig. 3) [11]. Marrow signal intensity alone cannot differentiate leukemic cells from cells of normal hematopoiesis, especially not in the younger age groups, in whom low signal intensity hematopoietic marrow can be seen. Therefore, calculated T1 relaxation times of marrow in the spine have been used to separate normal and abnormal marrow in children [7]. The T1 relaxation time of marrow is prolonged in children with newly diagnosed acute lymphocytic leukemia and in children in relapse, while the T1 marrow relaxation time of children in remission is similar to that of normal age-matched controls. The etiology of T1 prolongation is uncertain (decreasing fat content and increasing cellularity). Infiltration of the marrow by neoplastic cells other than leukemia (e.g. rhabdomyosarcoma, neuroblastoma) as well as hyperplasia of myeloid cells (e.g. *polycythemia vera*) also results in a prolongation of calculated T1 relaxation times [24].

Under therapy for leukemia, areas of *osteonecrosis* may develop. Therefore, MRI unexpectedly revealed bone marrow pathologies in children successfully treated for acute lymphoblastic leukemia, who had no symptoms [25]. In clinical routine MRI is used only exceptionally as a diagnostic method when leukemia is suspected. The diagnosis of relapse by MRI is only possible by performing MRI during the different stages of disease, especially clinical remission [26].

In vivo spectroscopy can be used to determine the relative percentage of fat and water protons within the marrow. In patients with leukemia the marrow shows a large water peak reflecting the presence of a cellular marrow. In response to treatment the water peak decreases and the fat peak increases [27-29].

Bone marrow myeloid depletion

It results from a loss of hematopoietic tissue. Causes are more acquired than congenital (infections, drugs, chemotherapy, radiation therapy, immune diseases). In these cases hematopoietic cells are decreased or are completely absent, fat cells occupy the marrow space. Aplastic or hypoplastic marrow shows a high-signal intensity on both T1- and T2-weighted images, reflecting replacement of red by yellow marrow. Foci of fibrosis can accompany the fatty replacement. In severe forms of anemias, fatty replacement is complete by 3 months. After treatment, regenerating red marrow is seen as focal or diffuse areas of decreased signal intensity on T1-weighted images [6, 7].

Myelofibrosis

It is characterized by replacement of the normal marrow cells by fibrotic tissue. In children this is usually the result of radiation therapy or chemotherapy for leukemia, lymphoma or metastatic disease. The fibrotic marrow shows bone-signal intensity on both T1- and T2-weighted images, whereas marrow infiltration of malignant cells is seen as intermediate-to-bright signal intensity on T2-weighted images [6, 7].

Post-therapy Alterations

Besides radiatin therapy and chemotherapy, *bone marrow transplantation* is another form of therapy used, e.g. for relapses of leukemia. The intravenously administered transplanted cells are engrafted within 3 to 4 weeks. The typical MR pattern of the vertebral marrow is usually seen within 90 days of transplantation. The T1-weighted images show a central zone of high intensity (fatty marrow) and a peripheral zone of intermediate signal intensity (repopulating hematopoietic marrow) [6, 7].

References

1. Foucar K (1995) Bone marrow pathology. American Society of Clinical Pathologists, ASCP Press, Chicago, pp 1-12
2. Vogler JB, Murphy WA (1988) Bone marrow imaging. Radiology 168: 679-693
3. Custer RP, Ahlfeldt FE (1932) Studies on the structure and function of bone marrow: II. Variations in cellularity in various bones with advancing years of life and their relative response to stimuli. J Lab Clin Med 17: 960-962
4. Custer RP (1932) Studies on the structure and function of

bone marrow: I. Variability of the hemopoietic pattern and consideration of methods for examination. J Lab Clin Med 10: 951-959

5. Kricun ME (1985) Red-yellow marrow conversion: its effects on the location of some solitary bone lesions. Skeletal Radiol 14: 10-19

6. Siegel MJ, Luker GD (1996) Bone marrow imaging in children. MRI Clin North Am 4: 771-796

7. Moore SG (1992) Pediatric musculoskeletal imaging. In: Stark DD, Bradley WG, JR (ed) MRI, 2nd edn. Mosby Year Book, St. Louis, Baltimore Boston Chicago London Philadelphia Sydney Toronto, pp 2223-2330

8. Hernandez RJ, Teo E-LHJ (1998) Diffuse marrow disorders in children. Magn Reson Imaging Clin N Am 6: 605-626

9. Jaramillo D, Laor T, Hoffer FA, Zaleske DJ, Cleveland RH, Buchbinder BR, Egglin TK (1991) Epiphyseal marrow in infancy: MR imaging. Radiology 180: 809-812

10. Jaramillo D, Connolly SA, Mulkern RV, Shapiro F (1998) Developing epiphysis: MR imaging characteristics and histologic correlation in the newborn lamb. Radiology 207: 637-645

11. Bohndorf K, Benz-Bohm G, Gross-Fengels W, Berthold F (1990) MRI of the knee region in leukemic children. Part I: initial pattern in patients with untreated disease. Pediatr Radiol 20: 179-183

12. Waitches G, Zawin JK, Poznanski AK (1994) Sequence and rate of bone marrow conversion in the femora of children as seen on MR imaging: are accepted standards accurate? AJR 162: 1399-1406

13. Moore DG, Dawson KL (1990) Red and yellow marrow in the femur: age-related changes in the appearance at MR imaging. Radiology 175: 219-223

14. Ricci C, Cova M, Kang YS, Yang A, Rahmouni A, Scott Jr. WW, Zerhouni EA (1990) Normal age-related patterns of cellular and fatty bone marrow distribution in the axial skeleton: MR imaging study. Radiology 177: 83-88

15. Dawson KL, Moore SG, Rowland JM (1992) Age-related marrow changes in the pelvis: MR and anatomic findings. Radiology 183: 47-51

16. Mankad VN, Williams JP, Harpen MD, Manci E, Longenecker G, Moore RB, Shah A, Yang YM, Brogdon BG (1990) Magnetic resonance imaging of bone marrow in sickle cell disease: clinical, hematologic, and pathologic correlations. Blood 75: 274-283

17. Rao VM, Mitchell DG, Rifkin MD, Steiner RM, Burk Jr. DL, Levy D, Ballas SK (1989) Marrow infarction in sickle cell anemia: correlation with marrow type and distribution by MRI. Magn Reson Imaging 7: 39-44

18. Rao VM, Mitchell DG, Steiner RM, Rifkin MD, Burk Jr. DL, Levy D, Ballas SK (1988) Femoral head avascular necrosis in sickle cell anemia: MR characteristics. Magn Reson Imaging 6: 661-667

19. Resnick D, Niwayama G (1995) Osteonecrosis: diagnostic techniques, specific situations, and complications. In: Resnick D (ed) Diagnosis of bone and joint disorders, 3rd edn. WB Saunders, Philadelphia, pp 3495-3558

20. Deely DM, Schweitzer ME (1997) MR imaging of bone marrow disorders. Radiol Clin North Am 35: 193-212

21. Levin TL, Sheth SS, Hurlet A, Comerci SC, Ruzal-Shapiro C, Piomelli S, Berdon WE (1995) MR marrow signs of iron overload in transfusion-dependent patients with sickle cell disease. Pediatr Radiol 25: 614-619

22. Levin TL, Sheth SS, Ruzal-Shapiro C, Abramson S, Piomelli S, Berdon WE (1995) MRI marrow observations in thalassemia: the effects of the primary disease, transfusional therapy, and chelation. Pediatr Radiol 25: 607-613

23. Papavasiliou C, Gouliamos A, Vlahos L, Trakadas S, Kalovidouris A, Pouliades GR (1990) CT and MRI of symptomatic spinal involvement by extramedullary haemopoiesis. Clin Radiol 42: 91-92

24. Jensen KE, Grube T, Thomsen C, Soerensen PG, Christoffersen P, Karle H, Henriksen O (1988) Prolonged bone marrow T_1-relaxation in patients with polycythemia. Magn Reson Imaging 6: 291-292

25. Ojala AE, Pääkkö E, Lanning FP, Harila-Saari AH, Lanning BM (1998) Bone marrow changes on MRI in children with acute lymphoblastic leukaemia 5 years after treatment. Clin Radiol 53: 131-136

26. Benz-Bohm G, Gross-Fengels W, Bohndorf K, Gückel C, Berthold F (1990) MRI of the knee region in leukemic children. Part II: follow up: responder, non responder, relapse. Pediatr Radiol 20: 272-276

27. Jensen KE, Jensen M, Grundtvig P, Thomsen C, Karle H, Henriksen O (1990) Localized in vivo proton spectroscopy of the bone marrow in patients with leukemia. Magn Reson Imaging 8: 779-789

28. Ballon D, Jakubowski A, Gabrilove J, Graham MC, Zakowski M, Sheridan C, Koutcher JA (1991) In vivo measurements of bone marrow cellularity using volume-localized proton NMR spectroscopy. Magn Reson Med 19: 85-95

29. Schick F, Einsele H, Weiß B, Forster J, Lutz O, Kanz L, Claussen CD (1996) Assessment of the composition of bone marrow prior to and following autologous BMT and PBSCT by magnetic resonance. Ann Hematol 72: 361-370

Malignant Tumors of the Dia/metaphysis

D. Jaramillo

Department of Radiology, Children's Hospital and Harvard Medical School, Boston, USA

Bone Tumors in the Pediatric Population

There are two main types of skeletal malignancies in children: round cell tumors and tumors that arise from mesenchymal elements [1]. Round cell tumors infiltrate the marrow, whereas mesenchymal tumors arise in areas of active ossification of cartilage and deposition of new bone. Marrow-infiltrating tumors include metastatic neuroblastoma, Ewing sarcoma, lymphoma, and Langerhans cell histiocytosis. All round cell tumors follow the distribution of hematopoietic bone marrow and do not produce tumor matrix. They destroy bone and are thus radiographically lytic. They also, however, elicit periosteal bone deposition and reactive bone formation both of which can increase radiographic density. Tumors related to the formation of cartilage and bone include osteogenic sarcomas, and cartilaginous tumors. These tumors tend to occur in the vicinity of the fastest growing physes (distal femur, proximal tibia, proximal humerus), and produce characteristic tumor matrix.

The incidence of bone neoplasms in children is age-related. Metastatic neuroblastoma is the most frequent cause of tumoral bone destruction in children under five years of age. Ewing sarcoma is the most common bone malignancy in children 5 to 10 years of age, whereas osteogenic sarcoma is the most common in adolescents [2].

Diagnosis of Malignant Bone Tumors

A skeletal malignancy in a child is suspected when a lesion has rapid growth or aggressive behavior. Most malignant masses are large at the time the patient seeks consultation. On radiographs, indistict (permeative or moth-eaten) borders, cortical destruction, a soft-tissue mass, tumor bone formation, aggressive periosteal reaction, and absence of bone remodeling suggest malignancy. This suspicion is heightened on cross-sectional images when the lesion has little or no perilesional edema, when the mass extends through the physis or into the joint, when there is invasion of the adjacent muscula-

ture, or when the adjacent vessels are markedly displaced or encased.

Once the initial evaluation suggests that the child may have a skeletal malignancy, the imaging evaluation should be directed towards guiding therapy. The main goals of imaging are: a) to determine local extent; b) to detect metastatic disease; c) to assess response to therapy; and d) to detect complications [3].

Local Extent

The assessment of local extent of the lesion is best done with MR imaging. The longitudinal extent of the tumor is of great importance to plan surgical therapy. In order to evaluate the length of the lesion, images with a large field of view must be done. T1-weighted images correlate better than other sequences with the extent of the lesion determined pathologically. The T1-weighted images are also useful to detect skip lesions and metastases or multifocal disease in the contralateral extremity [4].

Higher resolution longitudinal images are important to determine involvement of the epiphysis and joint space. Malignant lesions often violate the physis. Subperiosteal extension usually stops at the strong perichondral attachments. Extension into the joint is uncommon. In the knee, the site of 70% of osteosarcomas, extension is usually extrasynovial, along the cruciate ligaments [5]. Infrequently the synovium is invaded; in these cases the synovium is thick, nodular and very vascular, and there is usually a large effusion. Extension of tumor through articular cartilage is extremely rare.

On axial images, it is important to determine whether the lesion arises in the medullary cavity, in the surface of the bone, or in the soft tissues. Surface osteosarcomas and Ewing sarcomas have better prognosis than the central tumors. Primitive neuroectodermal tumors often arise from the soft tissues. The involvement of the vessels (particularly the popliteal vessels) and of the adjacent musculature is also very important for planning.

The dimensions of the tumor should be measured in the orthogonal planes. To increase reliability and reproducibility, we measure the images electronically and film the images displaying the measurements. More sophisticated volume determination and three dimensional rendering of the lesion are possible. Unfortunately, they are still laborious and time consuming. For planning of surgery or radiation therapy, it is important to calculate the distance between the tumor and the nearest articular surface, and between the tumor and the adjacent physis [3].

Metastatic Disease

Ninety per cent of malignant bone tumors in children are osteosarcomas and Ewing sarcomas (if we use this term to include primitive neuroectodermal tumors as well) [6]. The remainder are mostly cases of lymphoma, leukemia and metastatic neuroblastoma. Osteosarcoma and Ewing sarcoma have very similar patterns of metastatic spread: both tumors have frequent lung metastases, and both can have skeletal metastases. Evaluation of pulmonary metastasis requires chest CT, as the pulmonary lesions are usually small and difficult to detect radiographically. Any small nodule in the lung of a child is metastatic until proven otherwise. Since children tolerate thoracotomies well, and since the resection of pulmonary metastases improves survival, almost all nodules seen on CT are resected [7].

Prognosis of a bone tumor worsens significantly with the detection of bony metastases. Skeletal metastases are evaluated with ^{99m}Tc-methylene diphosphonate scintigraphy [8, 9]. The lesions are usually metaphyseal, but they can be seen anywhere in the skeleton. Extraskeletal metastases of osteosarcoma usually result in increased radiotracer uptake because they are bone forming.

Evaluation of Biologic Activity and Response to Therapy

Response to chemotherapy or radiation therapy can be evaluated with imaging by determining a decrease in size or biologic activity. The assessment of response based on tumoral size has several limitations. On MR images, the signal intensity of the involved marrow almost never returns to normal, even after complete tumor necrosis [3, 10]. Furthermore, tumoral death often results in the development of areas of cystic necrosis or hemorrhage, both of which can enlarge the size of the tumor mass. If the mass does decrease in size on axial images, or if there is marked decrease in enhancement, the tumor is presumed to be undergoing necrosis [11].

The advent of dynamic gadolinium-enhanced MR imaging has contributed significantly to the evaluation of tumor necrosis [12] and the differentiation of tumor versus edema [13]. With this technique, multiple images with a temporal resolution under 3 seconds are obtained before and after the administration of gadolinium. The rate of enhancement of each pixel and the characteristics of the enhancement curve can be analyzed. A "slope"-weighted image can be generated where the signal intensity of each pixel represents the slope of the enhancement curve. Granulation tissue and peritumoral edema have a slower rate of enhancement than active tumor [14]. Dynamic imaging can also help in differentiating benign from malignant soft-tissue masses, but is not sensitive or specific for differentiating benign from malignant bone tumors [15].

Thallium-201 (^{201}Tl) scannning is used with increasing frequency for the evaluation of active tumor in osteogenic sarcomas [16]. The tumoral uptake of thallium is a reflection of the vascularity, cellular viability and metabolic activity of the lesion. Following chemotherapy, responders show a marked decrease in tumoral uptake, whereas non-responders show no change or an increase in uptake [17-19].

More recently, positron emission tomography (PET) scanning has proven to be a very effective method to assess tumor viability and metastatic disease [20].

Osteogenic Sarcoma

Osteogenic sarcoma is the most frequent primary malignant tumor of bone in childhood. It affects children in the second decade of life; only 21% of affected children are younger than 10 years [21]. Although most cases are idiopathic, osteogenic sarcoma can develop after radiotherapy (usually 10 or more years after therapy), generally for a prior Ewing sarcoma. Children with hereditary retinoblastoma have a strong predisposition to osteogenic sarcoma [22].

Osteogenic sarcoma occurs most frequently in the metaphyses of fast growing bones such as the distal femur (40%), proximal tibia (20%), and proximal humerus (15%) [1, 23]. When imaging, it is important to determine whether there is extension into the epiphysis, which is detectable by MR imaging in 80% of cases [24]. It is also important to detect intra-articular extension, which is almost always extrasynovial [5]. Involvement of the neurovascular bundle (particularly the popliteal vessels) or major muscle groups such as the quadriceps may preclude limb-salvage surgery [25].

Ewing Sarcoma and Primitive Neuroectodermal Tumor of Bone

Ewing sarcoma and the closely related primitive neuroectodermal tumor (PNET) of bone constitute the second most common primary bone tumor of childhood. Ewing sarcoma and PNET are now considered to be the same tumor with variable differentiation, defined by a translocation between the *EWS* gene on chromosome 22 with an *ETS*-like gene, usually the *FLI-1* gene on chromosome 11 [26]. The two lesions are indistinguishable radiographically [27] and on histological examination both are composed of small, round cells, probably of neural origin [28]. Ewing sarcoma can resemble osteomyelitis and any other round-cell tumor of childhood such as metastatic neuroblastoma and lymphoma [29].

In more than half of the cases Ewing sarcoma inolves the extremities. The tumor is also commonly seen in the pelvis. The tumor is commonly thought of as being diaphyseal; the most common location, however, is the metaphysis (45%), and only one third of Ewing sarcomas involve the diaphysis. The lesions in the diaphysis are usually central, whereas those in the metaphysis are eccentric [30]. Periosteal reaction, in lamina parallel to the cortex (onion skin) or spiculated perpendicular to the cortex is seen in 60% of patients [31, 32]. Soft tissue masses are seen in 80% of cases.

Conclusion

Radiology has an increasingly important role in the management of musculoskeletal malignancies in children. Diagnostic imaging has become essential in defining the severity of the lesion, planning therapy, and in assessing the response to therapy.

References

1. Resnick D, Kyriakos M, Greenway GD (1995) Tumors and tumor-like lesions of bone: imaging and pathology of specific tumors. In: Resnick D (ed) Diagnosis of bone and joint disorders, 3rd edn. WB Saunders, Philadelphia, pp 3662-3697
2. Meyer JS, Dormans JP (1998) Differential diagnosis of pediatric musculoskeletal masses. Magn Reson Imaging Clin N Am 6: 561-577
3. Jaramillo D, Laor T, Gebhardt MC (1996) Pediatric musculoskeletal neoplasms. Evaluation with MR imaging. Magn Reson Imaging Clin N Am 4: 749-770
4. Laor T, Chung T, Hoffer FA, Jaramillo D (1996) Musculoskeletal magnetic resonance imaging: how we do it. Pediatr Radiol 26: 695-700
5. Schima W, Amann G, Stiglbauer R, et al. (1994) Preoperative staging of osteosarcoma: efficacy of MR imaging in detecting joint involvement. AJR 163: 1171-1175
6. Fletcher BD (1991) Response of osteosarcoma and Ewing sarcoma to chemotherapy: imaging evaluation. AJR 157: 825-833
7. Goorin AM, Shuster JJ, Baker A, et al. (1991) Changing pattern of pulmonary metastases with adjuvant chemotherapy in patients with osteosarcoma: results from the Multi-institutional Osteosarcoma Study. J Clin Oncol 9: 600-605
8. Goldstein H, McNeil B, Zufall E, Jaffe N, Treves S (1980) Changing indications for bone scintigraphy in patients with osteosarcoma. Radiology 135: 177-180
9. Rees C, Siddiqui A, duCret R (1986) The role of bone scintigraphy in osteogenic sarcoma. Skeletal Radiol 15:365-367
10. Lang P, Johnston JO, Arenal-Romero F, Gooding CA (1998) Advances in MR imaging of pediatric musculoskeletal neoplasms. Magn Reson Imaging Clin N Am 6: 579-604
11. Holscher H, Bloem J, Vanel D, et al. (1992) Osteosarcoma: chemotherapy-induced changes at MR imaging. Radiology 182: 839-844
12. Ma LD, McCarthy EF, Bluemke DA, Frassica FJ (1998) Differentiation of benign from malignant musculoskeletal lesions using MR imaging: pitfalls in MR evaluation of lesions with a cystic appearance. AJR 170: 1251-1258
13. Lang P, Honda G, Roberts T, et al. (1995) Musculoskeletal neoplasm: perineoplastic edema versus tumor on dynamic postcontrast MR images with spatial mapping of instantaneous enhancement rates (see comments) (published erratum appears in Radiology 1996 198: 910-911). Radiology 197: 831-839
14. Fletcher B, Hanna S, Fairclough D, Gronemeyer S (1992) Pediatric musculoskeletal tumors: use of dynamic, contrast-enhanced MR imaging to monitor response to chemotherapy. Radiology 184: 243-248
15. van der Woude HJ, Verstraete KL, Hogendoorn PC, Taminiau AH, Hermans J, Bloem JL (1998) Musculoskeletal tumors: does fast dynamic contrast-enhanced subtraction MR imaging contribute to the characterization? Radiology 208: 821-828
16. Menendez L, Fideler B, Mirra J (1993) Thallium-201 scanning for the evaluation of osteosarcoma and soft tissue sarcoma. J Bone Joint Surg 75: A526-A531
17. Caluser C, Abdel-Dayem H, Macapinlac H, et al. (1994) The value of thallium and three-phase bone scans in the evaluation of bone and soft tissue sarcomas. Eur J Nucl Med 21: 1198-1205
18. Ramanna L, Waxman A, Binney G, et al. (1990) Thallium-201 scintigraphy in bone sarcoma: comparison with gallium-67 and technetium-99m MDP in the evaluation of chemotherapeutic response. J Nucl Med 31: 567-572
19. Rosen G, Loren G, Brien E, et al. (1993) Serial thallium-201 scintigraphy in osteosarcoma. Correlation with tumor necrosis after preoperative chemotherapy. Clin Orthop 293: 302-306
20. Tse N, Hoh C, Hawkins R, Phelps M, Glaspy J (1994) Positron emission tomography of pulmonary metastases in osteogenic sarcoma. Am J Clin Oncol 17: 22-25
21. Parker B, Castellino R (1997) Pediatric oncologic radiology. Mosby, St. Louis
22. Link MP, Eilber F (1993) Osteosarcoma. In: Pizzo PA, Poplack DG (eds) Pediatric oncology. J.B. Lippincott, Philadelphia, pp 841-866
23. Mirra JM (1989) Bone tumors. Lea & Febiger, Philadelphia
24. Norton K, Hermann G, Abdelwahab I, Klein M, Granowetter L, Rabinowitz J (1991) Epiphyseal involvement in osteosarcoma. Radiology 180: 813-816
25. Springfield DS (1991) Introduction of limb-salvage surgery for sarcomas. Orthop Clin North Am 22: 1-17
26. Grier HE (1997) The Ewing family of tumors. Ewing's sarcoma and primitive neuroectodermal tumors. Pediatr Clin North Am 44: 991-1004
27. Eggli K, Quiogue T, Moser RJ (1993) Ewing's sarcoma. Radiol Clin North Am 31: 325-337
28. Horowitz ME, DeLaney TE, Malawer MM, Tsokos MG (1993) Ewing's sarcoma family of tumors: Ewing's sarcoma of bone and soft tissue and the peripheral primitive neuroectodermal tumors. In: Pizzo PA, Poplack DG (eds) Pediatric oncology. J.B. Lippincott, Philadelphia, pp 795-821
29. Mirra JM (1989) Bone tumors: Ewing's sarcoma. Lea & Febiger, Philadelphia, pp 143-438
30. Sherman R, Soong K (1956) Ewing's sarcoma: its roentgen classification and diagnosis. Radiology 66: 529-539

31. Reinus WR, Gilula LA, Committee I (1984) Radiology of
    Ewing's Sarcoma: Intergroup Ewing's Sarcoma Study. Radi-
    ographics 4: 929-944
32. Reinus W, Gilula L, Donaldson S, Shuster J, Glicksman A,
    Vietti T (1993) Prognostic features of Ewing sarcoma on
    plain radiograph and computed tomography scan after initial
    treatment. A Pediatric Oncology Group study (8346). Can-
    cer 72: 2503-2510

SESSION IV

SESSION IV

Imaging of the Postsurgical Pediatric Abdomen

A. Daneman

Department of Diagnostic Imaging, The Hospital for Sick Children, University of Toronto, Toronto, Canada

Introduction

Following any abdominal surgery, changes in the tissues at the site of the incision as well as within the abdominal cavity are to be expected as a normal response to the trauma and changes created by the surgery. These have to be differentiated from those unexpected changes or complications related to the surgery, which usually require medical or further surgical intervention.

Expected Changes

At the site of the wound incision and at the site of surgery within the abdomen (i) soft tissue swelling due to edema and (ii) collections of air are common findings. Imaging in the immediate postoperative period has to differentiate these normal findings from infectious complications or possible residual tumours (Fig. 1). At these sites there may also be small (iii) fluid collections or small hematomas and the child's clinical status may dictate whether any intervention is required.

It has been shown on plain radiographs that free intra-abdominal air will have disappeared by the second postoperative day in newborns and by the third postoperative day in most older children. However, in older children with small abdominal incisions (e.g. McBurney) some free intra-abdominal air may persist for 8 days and in those with larger incisions may even persist in a few patients until 3 weeks postoperatively.

Gastrointestinal function (peristalsis) (iv) may come to a temporary halt (ileus) producing gaseous distention, nausea and vomiting after most intra-abdominal operations. This occurs for several reasons including handling of the gastrointestinal tract or adjacent organs during surgery, pain and drugs. The degree to which this ileus occurs will depend on the type of operation and usually gastric peristalsis will take a few days to return, the small bowel peristalsis will usually return within 24 h and colonic motility after 48-72 h. Because the pediatric patient swallows considerable air the postoperative ileus may be prolonged in some patients.

Following removal of viscera or abdominal masses the remaining viscera will usually shift in position and there is a pattern of shift that can be recognized and is

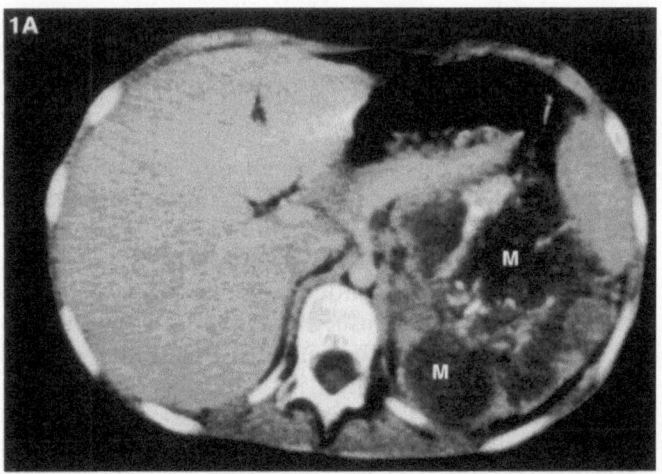 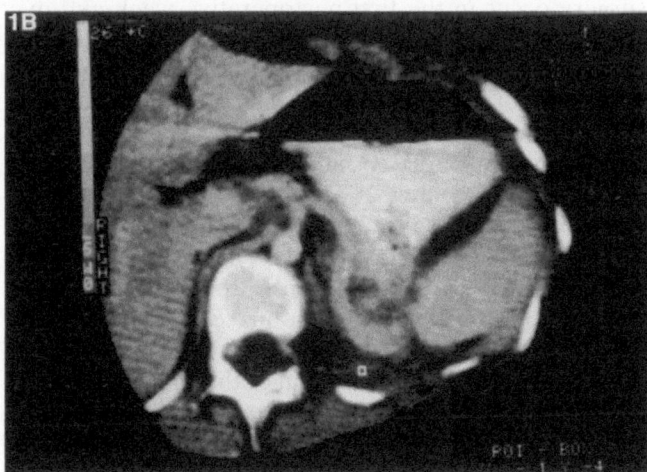

Fig. 1. a 12-year-old girl with masculinization due to large left adrenal carcinoma (M). **b** Postoperatively the mass has been completely removed but some soft tissue thickening (square cursor) outlines some postoperative change due to edema

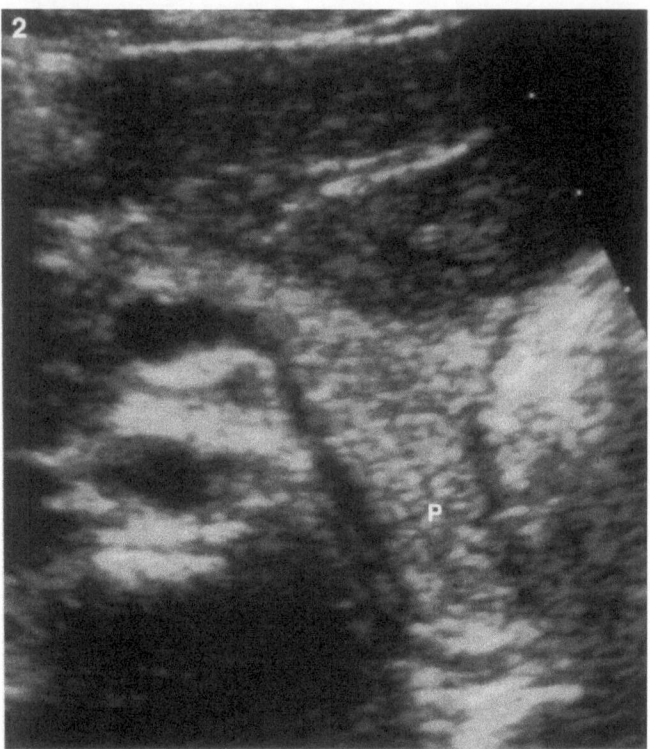

Fig. 2 Transverse sonogram of the upper abdomen following removal of left Wilm's tumour shows pancreatic tail (P) lying in left renal bed

to be expected (v). For example, following right nephrectomy the small and large bowel may fill the renal fossa and following left nephrectomy the bowel and the pancreatic tail may fill the left renal fossa (Fig. 2).

Complications

The vast majority of complications following abdominal surgery occur in the first postoperative week and may develop as (i) a direct result of the surgery itself; (ii) a result of the disease that had required the surgery; or (iii) for other unrelated causes. Whatever the reason the pediatric surgeon must be aware of the causes, must recognize them immediately, and must correct them as they arise. Clinical confirmation alone of the presence of such complications is not always possible and in this regard the pediatric radiologist plays a major role in imaging the postoperative abdomen with various modalities in an attempt to document the presence or absence of any complications and to differentiate significant findings from the more minor changes that have been mentioned above.

Soft Tissue Swelling and Fluid

Abnormal amounts of soft tissue swelling or fluid col-

lections either at the site of the incision or within the abdomen are highly suggestive of either infection or hematoma. Bleeding following surgery is indeed quite rare and the commonest cause for free or focal fluid collections is due to infection with or without abscess formation. The presence of fever toward the end of the first week after laparotomy strongly suggests a wound infection. A deep infection may not be clinically evident for several more days. Wound infection may be easily recognized clinically but persistent or spiking fever should raise the suspicion of an intra-abdominal abscess. Although sonography may depict most abscesses accurately and clearly, computed tomography may be necessary in those children with more extensive abscess collections in order to define the smaller locules and interloop components more accurately, particularly when percutaneous aspiration and drainage is required. Interventional radiology has come to play a major role in this clinical setting. Any focus of infection in or outside the abdominal cavity may prolong the postoperative ileus until the infection is adequately controlled. Spreading cellulitis, necrotizing fasciitis and wound dehiscence are uncommon complications.

Mechanical Bowel Obstruction

The postoperative ileus usually resolves by the first day in children but may be prolonged in the presence of electrolyte imbalance or focal or general sepsis. Occasionally a postoperative ileus may blend imperceptibly into postoperative mechanical obstruction, which usually requires nasogastric tube decompression. If the bowel obstruction is adhesive in nature, resolution of the fibrous adhesions will usually occur spontaneously in time. However, one must always consider an unusual cause of mechanical bowel obstruction in the postoperative period and this is the rare postoperative intussusception. This almost always follows 1-2 weeks after a major laparotomy and usually involves only the small bowel. There is seldom rectal bleeding or a palpable mass and the diagnosis may be quite difficult clinically because of the nonspecific presentation. Sonography is usually diagnostic but the recognition of a small bowel intussusception in this clinical setting may be more difficult than the recognition of the usual idiopathic ileocolic intussusception (Fig. 3). The reason for this is that in the postoperative period, the small bowel will be distended from the mechanical obstruction and the intussusception in the small bowel often lies deep in the abdomen (deep to the dilated loops) and is smaller than ileocolic intussusception. Surgery is invariably required to reduce postoperative intussusception.

The risk of adhesive bowel obstruction following abdominal surgery is approximately 5% and over 80% of such cases develop within 2 years of the initial opera-

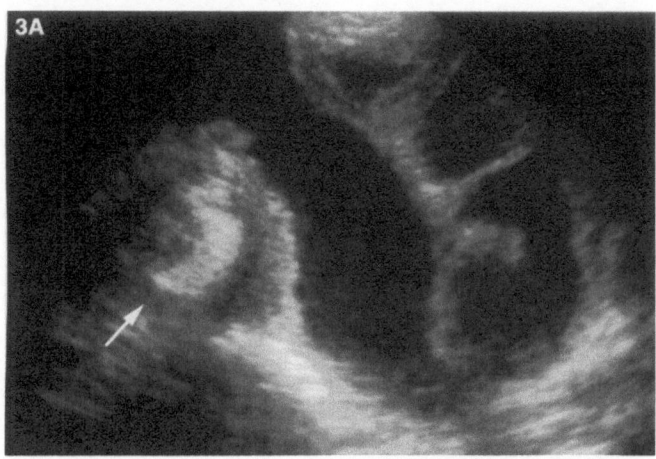 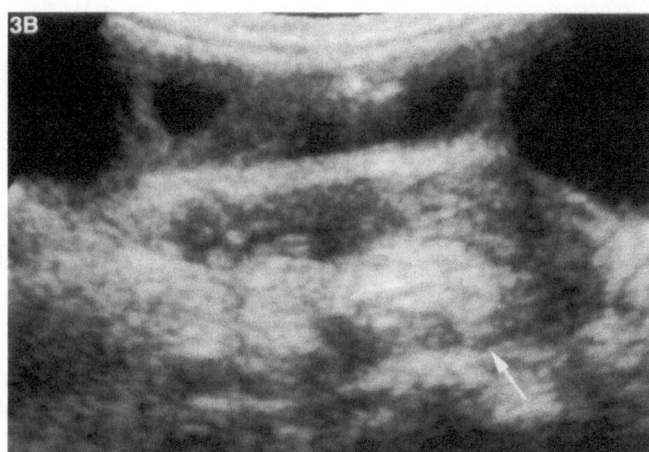

Fig. 3 a, b. Sonograms following laparotomy for removal of Wilm's tumour. This patient developed postoperative mechanical bowel obstruction due to a postoperative small bowel intussusception (arrows) shown in transverse in **a** and longitudinally in **b**

tion. It occurs most commonly in patients following laparotomy for inflammatory or neoplastic disease within the abdomen. Other causes of mechanical bowel obstruction to be considered include focal volvulus or internal hernia and these may be depicted on imaging modalities.

Unusual Visceral Shift

Following resection of viscera or masses the remaining viscera will move in to fill the space vacated and recognition of the usual movements described in the preceding text will exclude the presence of complications or recurrence of tumour. However, unusual visceral shifts may simulate the appearance of postoperative fluid collections or tumour recurrence on cross-sectional imaging (Fig. 4). The correct interpretation of the findings may become more difficult when

attention to meticulous technique fails to outline the viscera adequately. The use of posterior abdominal imaging in the prone position will facilitate imaging of the retroperitoneum and renal bed with sonography; adequate outline of the gastrointestinal tract with fluid or contrast agents will also be of value for defining the position of bowel on computed tomography scan.

Other Complications

Rare complications may be a direct result of complications of the surgery or the disease process and may include urinary and biliary obstruction as well as anastomotic leaks. Retention of surgical instruments and equipment is usually easily documented on plain radiographs but cross-sectional imaging may be required.

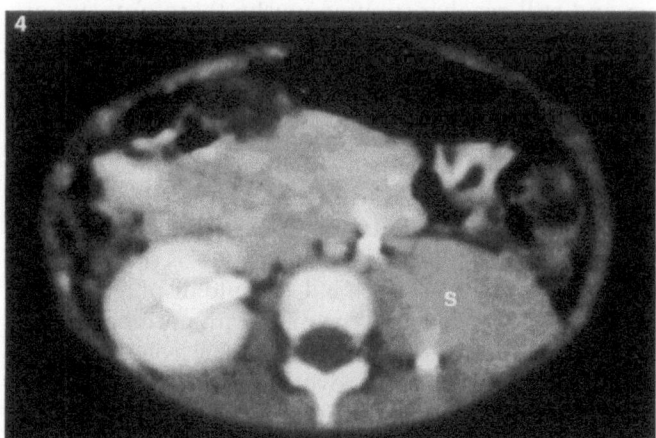

Fig. 4 Computed tomography scan following removal of left adrenal carcinoma and left kidney shows the spleen (S) lying in the left renal fossa. Surgical clips are seen anteriorly and posteriorly

Suggested Reading

Ein SH, Stephens CA, Reilly BJ (1985) The disappearance of free air after pediatric laparotomy. J Pediatr Surg 20: 422-424

Ein SH, Ferguson JM (1982) Intussusception: the forgotten postoperative obstruction. Arch Dis Child 57: 788-790

Janik JS, Ein SH, Filler RM, Shandling B, Simpson JS, Stephens CA (1981) An assessment of the surgical treatment of adhesive small bowel obstruction in infants and children. J Pediatr Surg 16: 225-229

Lang I, Connolly B, Daneman A (1997) An unusual position of the gallbladder following nephrectomy for large neoplasms. Pediatr Radiol 27: 528-529

Rowe MI, Tagge EP (1993) Pediatric physiology. In: Greenfield LJ, Mulholland MW, Oldham KT, Zelenock GB (eds) Surgery: scientific principles and practice. Lippincott, Philadelphia, pp 1791-1796

Wales PM, Murphy JJ, Janzen R, Gow K (1998) Adhesive small bowel obstruction in children: predictors of outcome. J Pediatr Surg (in press)

Right Lower Quadrant Pathology Including the Right Pelvis in the Pubertal Female

E.F. Avni[1], F. Ziereisen[1], M. Dassonville[2], N. Damry[1], C. Christophe[1], V. Segers[3]

[1]Departments of Medical Imaging, [2]Pediatric Surgery, [3]and Pathology, University Children's Hospital Queen Fabiola, Brussels, Belgium

Introduction

Pain in the right lower quadrant (RLQ) is common in children and represents a daily challenge for the clinician. This is even more difficult in the adolescent girl as the pain may have a gynecologic origin; furthermore, in girls, the psychological aspects are as important as the disease itself since their gynecologic future might be compromised.

Imaging plays an important role in helping the clinician to sort out the wide spectrum of diagnoses; among the techniques, ultrasound (US) is the main and sometimes the only tool necessary in order to study the anatomy and the changes caused by the disease.

The questions that have to be answered are:
- Is it the ovary (or another part of the reproductive organs) that is causing pain?
- Is it the appendix?
- What else could it be?

For each question, another presents itself: is surgical exploration mandatory?

Is it the Ovary?

In girls with RLQ pain diseases of the ovary and of the Fallopian tube represent the main differential diagnosis to appendicitis. Their evaluation should therefore be included in all examinations. One should not forget that many changes occur in these organs before, during and after puberty. This area is best studied by pelvic US; the examination should be performed using a high resolution sector transducer through a reasonably full bladder; some radiologists advocate a transvaginal approach, but this can only be performed in sexually active patients; this means that the sonologist must have a complete knowledge of the patient's history and that the examination must be performed under appropriate conditions.

Between the ages of 7 and 12 years, the ovaries and uterus develop progressively. The ovarian diameter increases from 1.5 to 3 cm, its volume from 1 to 3 cc; follicles grow in number and size, although it should be stressed that even before the age of 7 years, the normal ovary contains small cystic structures. The uterus length increases from 2 to 4 cm; the body thickens and the endometrial stripe appears as an echogenic line. The organs are considered mature when the ovary measures more than 3 cc, when at least four follicles are present, and when the body/cervix ratio of the uterus is above 1.2. After puberty, cyclic changes occur at the level of the endometrium and prominant follicles will appear and disappear in relation to the hormonal cycles.

As mentioned, in the case of RLQ pain, the uterus and adnexae should be systematically examined and signs indicating a pathology on us include the presence of *a mass, visible Fallopian tube, utero-vaginal abnormalities* and, to a lesser extent, *pelvic effusion*.

An *adnexal mass* is usually ovarian unless the ovaries are seen independently. A detailed US analysis should be performed in order to better characterise the mass (cystic, complex or solid mass, septa, nodules, calcifications, limits, signs of extension). An ovarian cystic structure does not necessarily correspond to a neoplasm and does not mean immediate surgery. Often it represents an atypical follicle. Normal follicles may reach up to 7-8 cm and still resolve spontaneously; therefore, surgery should be postponed until control examinations have been performed; in such cases, the pain may be related to a rapidly increasing volume of the follicle, to hemorrhage, to rupture or to torsion. In the case of *hemorrhage*, the contents appear highly echogenic (pseudo-solid) and will change during time.

Ovarian torsion represents a challenging diagnosis; symptoms include acute pain and a mass is often palpated; yet both are non-specific. US could display a specific pattern: adnexal solid type mass with peripheral follicles, but other patterns may exist. The role of duplex and color Doppler is controversial; cases have been reported in which a Doppler signal was present within the twisted ovary, on the other hand, vascularization is difficult to demonstrate in ovaries containing large follicles or cysts.

If the mass does not resolve on control examinations, other *ovarian tumors* should be considered. Both benign and malignant tumors can be encountered in this age group, the most common being teratomas. Supplementary imaging modalities, such as CT or MRI, may be necessary in order to analyse the mass, its content and its limits or to demonstrate extra-tumoral extension. Preoperative evaluation should also include the contralateral side as 15-25% of the tumors are bilateral. All masses are not ovarian and other potential diagnoses should be considered such as urachal anomalies, mesenteric or duplication cysts, lymphangioma and digestive tumors.

Pelvic inflammatory disease (PID) is being diagnosed more and more frequently in adolescent girls; clinically, pain and hyperthermia are present; leukocytosis is common. Sonographically, the adnexa appears swollen, a dilated Fallopian tube is visible, an abscess may be demonstrated and free fluid is present in the cul-de-sac; Doppler is useful as it demonstrates increased vascularization with a low resistivity index.

Ectopic pregnancy represents an important differential diagnosis in sexually active adolescents. In straightforward cases US demonstrates a gestational sac outside the uterus containing a viable embryo, but an heterogeneous adnexal mass – corresponding to a blood clot – is the only sign in non-specific cases; decidual reaction at the level of the uterus may be the clue to the diagnosis.

Pelvic endometriosis is almost never diagnosed preoperatively by US although surgical series describe numerous cases and suggest that it can be found in 20% of the laparoscopic series; the only presentation that can be diagnosed by US is *endometrioma*, in which a cystic echogenic mass is found.

At the level of the uterus, some congenital anomalies such as *hematocolpos* or *duplication* may be detected after puberty only. In case of hematocolpos, the vagina is distended and filled with an echogenic fluid, the uterine cavity is distended to a lesser extent. Duplication and septation anomalies of the uterus are more difficult to diagnose unless the uterine hemicavity is distended; associated urinary tract malformations may be present.

Finally, in this age group, *pregnancy* can occur and the sonologist should be prepared for such a diagnosis.

Appendicitis and Bowel Disease

Appendicitis is one of the main causes of RLQ pain in children and adolescents, yet about 20% of appendices removed are normal. It represents the main clinical concern. The use of US has modified the approach to this sometimes difficult diagnosis. The role of US is not only to confirm the diagnosis in doubtful cases but also to suggest alternatives. A positive US diagnosis for appendicitis is based not only on an increased diameter (above 6 mm), but also on graded compression and on the demonstration of surrounding hyperechoic inflammed mesenteric fat. An appendicolith is a supplementary positive finding; fluid may be present in variable amounts. Perforated appendix and/or peritonitis may be missed and examination by US and abdominal CT is helpful in such difficult cases.

An abscess may collect in the Cul-de-Sac and be misinterpreted as an ovarian mass.

Enlarged mesenteric adenopathies may be present with or without appendicitis. Every effort should be made to demonstrate a normal appendix before a conclusion of *mesenteric adenitis* can be made, which corresponds to the main differential diagnosis. Enlarged but small adenopathies (above 5 mm) may be demonstrated in normal patients. Large adenopathies (above 10 mm), may be present in various conditions including mesenteric adenitis, pharyngitis, gastroenteritis and inflammatory bowel disease. In the latter, thickened bowel loops will be demonstrated, usually at the ileo-caecal region; aperistaltic thickened small bowel loops are encountered in case of regional enteritis (Crohn's disease), where thickened colon orients towards ulcerative or infectious colitis.

Abdominal lymphoma and *tuberculosis* represent difficult, but important, differential diagnoses.

Unusual Diagnoses

Unusual or unexpected diagnosis for RLQ pain include *right lower lobe pneumonia, hepatitis, urinary tract* or *gallbladder diseases* and psoas abscess. There are a few case reports of omental infarction or deep vein thrombosis that presented with RLQ pain. One should also not forget to consider lumbar spine or hip anomalies.

Conclusion

Ultrasound is the main "assistant" to the radiologist in the challenging differential diagnosis of RLQ pain. In adolescent girls a balance must be achieved between appendicitis and gynecologic disease through a complete US survey of both areas. A good knowledge of prepubertal and pubertal changes is mandatory when dealing with such patients.

Suggested Reading

Siegel MJ, Carel C, Sunatt S (1991) Ultrasonography of acute abdominal pain in children. JAMA 266: 1987-1989

Dickson JAS, Telfer J, Jones A, de Dombal T (1988) Acute abdominal pain in children. Scand J Gastroenterol 23 :43-46

Irvin TT (1989) Abdominal pain: a surgical audit of 1190 emergency admissions. Br J Surg 76: 1121-1125

Scholer SJ, Pituch K, Orr DP, Dittro RS (1996) Clinical outcomes of children with acute abdominal pain. Pediatrics 98: 680-685

Banrjee R, Laufer MR (1998) Reproductive disorders associated with pelvic pain. Semin Pediatr Surg 7: 52-61

Athea N (1998) Ultrasonography of the pelvis in adolescents. Ann Pediatr 45: 341-347

Weimersheiner P (1997) Non-operative causes of abdominal pain. Surg Clin North Amer 77: 1433-1454

Teele RL, Share JC (1992) US of the female pelvis in childhood and adolescence. Radiol Clin North Amer 30: 743-758

States LJ, Bellah RD (1996) Imaging of the pediatric female pelvis. Semin Roentgenol 31: 312-329

Barnewolt C (1998) Imaging techniques to assess the pelvis in young females. Semin Pediatr Surg 7: 73-81

Bellah RD, Rosenberg HH (1991) Transvaginal US in children's hospital. Pediatr Radiol 21: 570-574

Cohen HL, Bober SE, Bow SN (1992) Imaging the pediatric pelvis: the normal and abnormal genital tract and simulators of its disease. Urol Radiol 14: 273-278

Cohen HL, Eisenberg P, Mandel F, Haller JO (1992) Ovarian cysts are common in premenarchal girls: US of 101 children 2-12 years old. AJR 159: 89-91

Helmrath MA, Shin CE, Warner BW (1998) Ovarian cysts in the pediatric population. Semin Pediatr Surg 7: 19-28

Warner BW, Kulu JC, Bau LL (1992) Conservative management of large ovarian cysts in children: the value of serial pelvic US. Surgery 112: 749-755

Quillin SP, Siegel MJ (1994) Transabdominal color Doppler US of the painful adolescent ovary. J Ultrasound Med 13: 549-555

Stark JE, Siegel MJ (1994) Ovarian torsion in prepubertal and pubertal girls US findings. AJR 163: 1479-1482

Willms AB, Schlund JF, Meyer WR (1995) Endovaginal Doppler US in ovarian torsion. Ultrasound Obstet Gynecol 5: 129-132

Sunatt JT, Siegel MJ (1991) Imaging of pediatric ovarian masses. Radiographics 11: 533-548

Rigsby CK, Siegel MJ (1994) CT appearance of pediatric ovaries and uterus. JCAT 18: 72-76

Quillin SP, Siegel MJ (1992) CT features of benign and malignant teratomas in children. JCAT 16: 722-726

Lazar EZ, Stolar CJH (1998) Evaluation and management of pediatric solid ovarian tumors. Semin Pediatr Surg 7: 29-34

Blythe MJ (1998) Pelvic inflammatory disease in the adolescent population. Semin Pediatr Surg 7: 43-51

Kupesic S, Kurjak A, Palasik L, et al. (1995) The value of transvaginal color Doppler in the assessment of pelvic inflammatory disease. Ultras Med Biol 21: 733-738

Golden Neuhoff S, Cohen H (1989) Pelvic inflammatory disease in adolescents. J Pediatr 114: 138-143

Ammerman S, Shafer MA, Snyder D (1990) Ectopic pregnancy in adolescents: a clinical review for pediatricians. J Pediatr 117: 677-686

Tran ATB, Arensman R, Falteman KW (1987) Diagnosis and management of hydrohematocolpos syndromes. AJDC 141: 632-634

Shatjkers DR, Haller JO, Velcek FT (1991) Imaging of uterovaginal anomalies in the pediatric patients. Urol Radiol 13: 58-66

Vignault F, Filiatrault D, Brandt ML, et al. (1990) Acute appendicitis in children: evaluation with US. Radiology 176: 501-504

Sivit G, Newman KD, Boening DA, et al. (1992) Appendicitis: usefulness of US in diagnosis in a pediatric population. Radiology 185: 549-552

Sivit CJ, Newman KD, Chandra RS (1993) Visualization of enlarged mesenteric lymphnodes at US examination. Pediatr Radiol 23: 471-475

Watanabe M, Ishii E, Hirowatari Y, et al. (1997) Evaluation of abdominal lymphadenopathy in children by US. Pediatr Radiol 27: 860-864

Rao PM, Rhea JT, Novelline RA (1997) CT diagnosis of mesenteric adenitis. Radiology 202: 405-409

Faure C, Belarbi N, Mougenot JF, et al. (1997) US assessment of inflammatory bowel disease in children: comparison with ilecolonoscopy. J Pediatr 130: 147-151

Karak PK, Millmond SH, Neumann D, Yamase HT, Ramsby G (1998) Omental infarction: report of three cases and review of the literature. Abdom Imaging 23: 96-98

Davey MS, Cohen MD (1996) Imaging of GI malignancy in childhood. Radiol Clin North Amer 34: 717-741

Disantis DJ, Siegel MJ, Katz ME (1991) Simplified approach to umbilical remnant abnormalities. Radiographics 11: 59-66

Avni EF, Matos C, Diard F, Schulman CC (1998) Midline omphalovesical anomalies in children. Urol Radiol 10: 189-194

Schwarz DS, Keller MS (1997) Deep venous thrombosis as a cause of pelvic pain in children. J Ultrasound Med 16: 281-289

Cheah WK, King PA, Tan HL (1994) A review of pediatric cases of urinary tract calculi. J Pediatr Surgery 29: 701-705

The Wide Spectrum of Inflammatory Bowel Disease in Children

A. Lebenthal,[1] E. Lebenthal[2]

[1] Department of Surgery, Hadassah University Hospital, Ein Karem, Jerusalem, Israel
[2] Department of Paediatrics, Hadassah University Hospital, Mt. Scopus, Jerusalem, Israel

The inflammatory bowel diseases (IBD), Crohn's Disease (CD) and ulcerative colitis (UC) are chronic inflammatory diseases of the intestines with a combined prevalence of 200-300 per 100 000 persons in the industrialized world [1]. The peak frequency of new cases of CD in the pediatric population is during the mid to late teens with an age-specific incidence of 16 per 100 000 persons [2]. It was suggested that a threefold rise in the incidence of CD occurred between 1968 to 1983, which further increased to 4.4 fold between 1968 and 1988 [3]. In contrast, UC did not show an upward trend during the same period [3]. A positive family history is the most consistent risk factor for children with IBD (odds ratio 5.6) [4].

There is strong evidence from twin studies, familial risk data and segregation analyses that IBD, especially CD might be genetic [5]. CD and UC are considered complex genetic traits as inheritance does not follow any simple Mendelian models [6]. The degree of genetic clustering in siblings has been estimated at 36.5 for CD, 16.6 for UC and 24.7 for IBD [7]. The cross-disease relative risks are 3.85 for UC given a CD proband and 1:72 conversely [5], suggesting the presence of shared susceptibility genes between UC and CD. However, there is conflicting data on the susceptibility locus for IBD in different chromosomes. In the search for a susceptibility loci for IBD a genome-wide screen in 41 CD sibling pairs testing 270 markers with replication in a second panel of 71 pairs demonstrated evidence for linkage over a broad, pericentromeric region on chromosome 16 [8]. This region subsequently has been confirmed for CD but not UC. A separate genome wide screen of 89 sibling pairs [9] showed linkage to chromosome 12 and two other IBD loci with evidence suggestive of linkage to chromosomes 7 and 3p [10].

The number of affected relative pairs undergoing the initial genome screen suggests that additional loci might be identified through genome wide screening. A genome wide screen on 297 CD, UC or mixed relative pairs from 174 American families (37% Ashkenazis) showed two novel regions on chromosomes 1p and 3q with suggestive evidence for linkage, and report nominal evidence for linkage in 15 additional chromosomal regions [10]. In conclusion, there is evidence suggesting linkage in all IBD families in two susceptibility regions on chromosomes 1p and 3q, and confirmatory evidence for linkage in the pericentromeric region of chromosome 16, IBD 1 [8].

Crohn's Disease (CD) may involve any part of the gut, most frequently the terminal ileum and colon [11]. Bowel inflammation is transmural, discontinuous and may contain granulomas or be associated with intestinal or perianal fistulas. In contrast, in UC, the inflammation is continuous, limited to rectal and colonic mucosal layers and fistulas or granulomas are not observed [11]. Colonic involvement in 10% of cases does not have a definite CD or UC and is designated indeterminate colitis. Both diseases present extraintestinal inflammation of the joints, skin and eyes. The prevalence of IBD is increased with ankylosing spondylitis and sclerosing cholangitis [11].

Ulcerative colitis (UC) tends to run a more complicated course in children than in adults. There is a greater likelihood of pancolonic as compared to limited colonic involvement and increased chance for proximal extension of initially localized disease. Diagnosis is generally made when the patient is between 5 and 16 years of age, but onset during infancy has been described. Variability in the age of onset, extent of intestinal involvement, severity of intestinal symptoms and extraintestinal manifestations results in diverse patterns of clinical presentation that necessitate individualized approaches to therapy.

Most pediatric gastroenterologists have been of the opinion that young children with pancolitis were subject to a particularly difficult course; however, Gryboski [12] reported contrasting results in a group of 38 children with UC who were diagnosed at less than 10 years of age. Although 71% of these children had pancolitis, the majority had clinically mild (53%) or moderate (37%) disease. Only 2 children underwent colectomy during a 6.7 year follow-up period.

Michener and colleagues [13] observed that the frequency of colectomy in children with UC decreased significantly during the past two decades. Although 48% of children with UC underwent colectomy between 1955 and 1965, the rate fell to 26.2% between 1965 and 1974. This change undoubtedly reflects improved treatment (e.g., intravenous nutritional support, new 5-Amino salycilic acid derivatives, steroids, broad-spectrum antibiotics, and immunosuppressive drugs). In addition, the use of colonoscopy for cancer surveillance rather than performing "prophylactic colectomy" has become standard practice in many centers for children whose disease improves with medical therapy.

There are several concerns regarding pediatric IBD, in addition to the early presentation of the intestinal and extraintestinal manifestations; primarily growth failure and retarded sexual maturation. Another concern is extraintestinal manifestations such as arthritis which can masquerade as juvenile rheumatoid arthritis; growth failure as idiopathic growth failure or even anorexia nervosa before intestinal manifestations are recognized. As in other pediatric chronic diseases, the long term management of IBD is a challenge for those associated with the treatment.

Although 60% of children with UC present with mild diarrhea of insidious onset, with or without blood in the stools, 10% present with a fulminant colitis. In childhood, UC appears in one of three forms; the most common is the insidious onset of diarrhea and rectal bleeding, without fever or abdominal pain, with disease that remains confined to the distal colon. In the second type bloody diarrhea, tenesmus, urgency, low-grade fever, weight loss, and mild anemia are present. Physical findings generally are limited to abdominal tenderness. In severe disease, more than six bloody stools per day, tachycardia, weight loss, anemia, and hypoalbuminemia occur; abdominal examination reveals diffuse tenderness, but without peritoneal signs. Toxic megacolon is uncommon but if it exists it represents a true emergency situation [14].

Probably the most important aspect of diagnosing UC is the exclusion of entric infection. Pathogens that may nimic UC include *Salmonella*, *Shigella*, *Campylobacter*, *Aeromonas*, *Plesiomonas*, *Yersinia*, *Escherichia coli 0157:H7*, *Clostridium difficile*, and *Entamoeba histolytica*. In some cases, acute bacterial gastroenteritis may be associated with or trigger the first episode of IBD. Histologic features have been described that differentiate acute infectious colitis from IBD; however, based on reports in the literature, it may not always be possible to accurately distinguish an acute infectious process from UC early in the course of disease, even with an assessment of biopsy material.

Initial, screening tests should include stool examinations for enteric pathogens, occult blood and fecal leukocytes, and selected blood tests. The blood tests used for screening children for UC include complete blood count (with attention to detecting a reduced mean corpuscular volume and elevated band count, with or without leukocytosis), platelet count, serum albumin, erythrocyte sedimentation rate, and C-reactive protein. It was noted that thrombocytosis, hypoalbuminemia, and high serum oro-

somucoid correlate best with histologic inflammation of the colon in UC. Important to note, however, is that 36% of pediatric patients had no abnormal blood test results. Acute phase reactants (e.g., erythrocyte sedimentation rate, C-reactive protein, or orosomucoid) are more likely to be elevated in patients with CD than in those with UC. Radiologic assessment of skeletal age is indicated in children with unexplained short stature to determine whether delayed maturation is present.

In CD [15], periumbilical abdominal pain, which is colicky in nature and worse after meals, diarrhea, and weight loss are the most common presenting symptoms. The cause of diarrhea in patients with CD is multifactorial; extensive mucosal dysfunction, bile acid malabsorption in terminal ileal disease, bacterial overgrowth secondary to strictures and disordered motility, and protein exudation from inflamed surfaces lead to diarrhea. Rectal blood loss may be apparent with colitis. CD is often insidious in onset, and extraintestinal symptoms such as intermittent fever, arthritis, iridocyclitis, erythema nodosum, or growth retardation may predominate, with few or no symptoms that suggest gastrointestinal involvement. In children, malnutrition and abnormalities in growth often are present. With mild, short-term disease, the weight-for-height may be depressed; in severe disease, wasting may be extreme and hypoalbuminemia may be present. In chronic, long-term disease, children may be short in stature, but with a weight appropriate for their height. Anemia is present in as many as 50% of all patients. Not surprisingly, the initial diagnosis in affected children often is incorrect, and conversely, the correct diagnosis may be delayed considerably. In general, the average delay between the onset of symptoms and the diagnosis is 1 year. Moreover, delayed referral may raise this figure to nearly 3 years. The site and extent of disease have a considerable effect upon the delay in diagnosis; left-sided colonic disease (2 months) is diagnosed more rapidly than either diffuse small bowel disease (5 months) or disease confined to the terminal ileum and right colon (16 months). In children, ileocolitis is the most common (52%) and colitis (9%) is the least common form of disease, with diffuse small bowel disease and ileal involvement each accounting for about 20% of all cases. The importance of seeking diagnostic clues outside the abdomen cannot be overemphasized. Thus, the presence of clubbing, perianal disease including skin tags, fissures and fistula, oral ulceration, uveitis or arthritis provide valuable information on which a clinical diagnosis may be based [15].

Abdominal pain and diarrhea are present in the majority of affected children. The pain is commonly in the right lower quadrant and may be associated with tenderness on palpation together with a fullness or mass. Periumbilical or left-sided pain may also be observed. Recently, we have seen more patients with upper gastrointestinal involvement. In the presence of esophageal or gastroduodenal involvement, epigastric discomfort, often of a "dyspeptic" nature, may be noted. Frequently, the abdominal pain associated with CD is severe and may wake the child from sleep. Aphthus stomatitis and aphthoid lesions in the mouth are seen in some of the patients.

Diarrhea may be variable in severity, ranging from one to two loose stools daily to marked diarrhea (>6 stools/day), occurring both at night and during the day. Gross blood in the stool is more common with colonic than small bowel involvement, although deep small bowel ulceration may precipitate severe hemorrhage. Anorexia, nausea and vomiting are common. Perirectal disease (e.g., fistulae, fissures, and tags) are observed in approximately 15-30% of patients.

Systemic manifestations, such as fever, fatigue and weight loss are noted in a majority of patients. The most common extraintestinal manifestations are in the skin, joints, liver, eye and bone. Erythema nodosum is more common in CD than UC and usually reflects active bowel inflammation. In approximately 74% of patients in whom erythema nodosum develops, arthritis also develops. Pyoderma gangrenosum is rare in patients with CD.

Two forms of joint involvement may be observed, including a peripheral form called enteropathic synovitis or colitic arthritis; an axial form, including ankylosing spondylitis or sacroiliitis. The kees, ankles, and hips are the commonly involved peripheral joints. Because 50% of patients with IBD in whom arthritis develops also develop ocular inflammation, routine ophthalmologic evaluation is warranted. Hypertrophic osteoarthropathy or clubbing is noted in as many as 30% of patients.

Abnormal serum aminotransferases are noted in approximately 15% of children with IBD during their course. Transient elevations are frequently associated with disease flares; medications such as 6-mercaptopurine or sulfasalazine; parenteral hyperalimentation; and hepatic steatosis from corticosteroids, malnutrition, or massive weight gain. Two more serious chronic conditions that may arise include chronic active hepatitis and sclerosing cholangitis. These complications develop in less than 1% of all children with CD but may result in cirrhosis of the liver and liver failure.

Ocular complications are observed with other extraintestinal manifestations. Patients with colonic involvement are more likely than those with small bowel disease to develop uveitis, scleritis, or episcleritis. The chronic administration of high-dose daily corticosteroids may be complicated by the development of increased intraocular pressure and cataracts.

Diminished bone density has been reported in patients with CD at diagnosis and during the disease course. Factors that might be operative include poor diet with protein-calorie deprivation, inadequate calcium intake or malabsorption, vitamin D deficiency, excessive cytokine production by the inflamed bowel that interferes with bone metabolism, and corticosteroid inhibition of calcium absorption and direct inhibition of bone formation. Accelerated bone mineral loss may occur with prolonged bed rest and corticosteroid-induced hypercalciuria.

Additional extraintestinal complications are right-sided hydronephrosis in the setting of ileocolonic inflammation when an inflammation mass encases the right ureter, hypercoagulability with venous thrombosis, pancreatitis, autoimmune anemia, and vasculitis.

In 20% of children with CD, a decrease in growth velocity may precede overt gastrointestinal symptoms by months or years. Absolute height deficits are observed in as many as 40% of children, with almost 50% of patients having weight-for-age measurement less than 90% of those expected. Factors that have been proposed to contribute to poor growth in these children include chronic malnutrition, corticosteroid administration, and a still poorly defined growth-retarding effect of chronic inflammation. Malnutrition occurs because of suboptimal dietary intake, increased gastrointestinal losses, and malabsorption. Although most studies have not shown increased basal caloric requirements in patients with CD, factors such as fever may increase caloric demands. Anorexia is very common and is not always secondary to fear of precipitating gastrointestinal symptoms. A central appetite-reducing effect of circulating proinflammatory cytokines has been suggested but not proven. Delayed gastric emptying in some children may lead to early satiety.

Growth hormone levels have been found to be normal in children with growth delay secondary to CD. Serum insulin-like growth factor-1 (IGF-1) levels are low in most patients with growth abnormalities and likely reflect a poor nutritional state. IGF-binding protein 1 (IGF-BP 1) serum levels are similar in growth-retarded and normally growing children with CD.

Daily corticosteroid therapy may inhibit growth at several levels. Corticosteroids may inhibit the biologic activity of IGF-1, inhibit several steps in collagen synthesis, and promote negative calcium balance by decreasing intestinal absorption and increasing urinary loss. Alternate-day corticosteroid therapy, however, does not seem to inhibit growth. Serum levels of the C-terminal propeptide of type I collagen and the N-terminal propetide of type III collagen are significantly lower in children with slow growth velocity who are on daily corticosteroids, regardless of disease activity. However, it is often difficult to separate the relative contributions of disease activity from corticosteroid usage in the pathogenesis of slow linear growth. It should be emphasized that the eradication of gastrointestinal symptoms by high-dose daily corticosteroid therapy with the concomitant compromise of growth is not considered successful medical management.

The main aims of therapy for inflammatory bowel disease in children and adolescents are: [1] the induction and maintenance of remission; [2] the correction of nutrient deficits; and [3] the restoration of growth and maturation. These goals are reached with the use of a combination of therapeutic methods, including pharmacologic agents, nutritional and psychological support, and surgical intervention. The commonly used drugs 5-amino salicylate, derivatives, sulfasalazine, corticosteroids and metronidazole have all been shown to be safe and efficacious when given to children. Newer steroid preparations that are rapidly degraded either in the target issue or elsewhere are being suggested. Of these, budesonide shows promise as an efficacious drug with few side effects, but its use in children needs further study. Newer 5-amino-salicylate preparations such as Asacol and Pentasa have been shown to be effective in children. Immunomodulatory drugs such as azathioprine 6-mercaptopurine and cyclosporin A appear to be safe and efficacious for children; cyclosporine has been used infrequently to treat refractory CD in children. Recently, a new drug, tumor necrosis factor (TNF)-α antibody (Infliximab; Centocor Inc [16]) was recommended for patients with moderate to severe CD for whom conventional therapy is inadequate. The use of other agents such as methotrexate, tacrolimus, monoclonal antibodies to cytokines, antibiotics and specific dietary products such as fish oils have not been intensively studied in children with CD. Nutritional therapy remains a mainstay of treatment because it corrects nutritional deficits, replaces losses and stimulates growth.

References

1. Calkins BM, Mendeloff AI (1986) Epidemiology of inflammatory bowel disease. Epidemiol Rev 8: 60-91
2. Haug K, Schrump EH, Halverson JF, et al. and the study group of IBD in western Norway (1989) Epidemiology of Crohn's disease in western Norway. Scand J Gastroenterol 24: 1271
3. Barton RJ, Gillon S, Ferguson A (1989) Incidence of IBD in Scottish children between 1968 and 1983, marginal fall in UC, three fold rise in CD. Gut 30: 618
4. Gilat T, Hacohen D, Lios P, et al. (1987) Childhood factors in UC and CD. An international cooperative study. Scand J Gastroenterol 22: 1009
5. Orholm M, Munkholm P, Langholz E, Nielsen OH, Sorensen TIA, Binder V (1991) Familial occurrence of inflammatory bowel disease. J Engl J Med 324: 84-88
6. Lander ES, Schork NJ (1994) Genetic dissection of complex traits. Science 265: 2037-2048
7. Satsangi J, Jewell DP, Bell JI (1997) The genetics of inflammatory bowel disease. Gut 40: 572-574
8. Hugot JP, Laurent-Puig P, Gower-Rousseau C, Olson JM, Le JC, et al. (1966) Mapping of a susceptibility locus for Crohn's disease on chromosome 16. Nature 379: 821-823
9. Cho JH, Nicolae DL, Gold LH, et al. (1998) Identification of novel susceptibility loci for inflammatory bowel disease on chromosome 1 p, 3q and 4q: evidence for epitasis between 1 p and IBD1. Proc Natl Acad Sci 95: 7502-7507
10. Satsangi J, Parkes M, Louis E, et al. (1996) Two stage genome-wide search in inflammatory bowel disease provides evidence for susceptibility loci on chromosomes 3,7 and 12. Nat Genet 14: 199-202
11. Podolsky DK (1991) Inflammatory bowel disease. N Engl J Med 325: 928-937; 1008-1009
12. Gryboski JD (1993) Ulcerative colitis in children 10 years or younger. J Pediatr Gastroenterol Nutr 17: 24-31
13. Michener WM, Whelan G, Greenstreet RL, et al. (1982) Comparison of the clinical features of CD and UC with onset in childhood or adolescence. Clev Clin J Med 49: 13-16
14. Kirschner SB (1996) Ulcerative colitis in children. Pediatr Clin North Amer 43: 235-254
15. Hyams JS (1996) Crohn's disease in children. Pediatr Clin North Amer 43: 255-277
16. van Deventer SJ (1997) Tumor necrosis factor and Crohn's disease. Gut 40: 443-448

Testicular and Pelvic Tumors

M.D. Cohen

Department of Radiology, Indiana University School of Medicine, Indiana, USA

Introduction

The pelvis and testes are not uncommon sites for tumors in children [1]. Although the differential diagnosis for tumors in these sites is extremely large, most of these tumors fall into four types (Table 1).

Primary tumors of the testes are rare, about 1% of all childhood malignancies. Almost all primary tumors of the scrotum arise in the testes with the exception of rhabdomyosarcoma, which may arise in the testes or in the adjacent structures [2]. The classification of testicular tumors in children is given in Table 2.

Rhabdomyosarcoma in the Pelvis and Scrotum

Rhabdomyosarcoma arises from a primitive cell that has the potential for differentiating into muscle. Most rhabdomyosarcomas are found in sites where muscle is not normally located. Rhabdomyosarcoma can be found in virtually any organ or tissue in the body, and it has the most widespread distribution of any pediatric tumor. It is interesting and unusual because its behavior is unique for each different anatomic location. The etiology of the tumor is unknown and it does not have good biological markers. The tumor occurs most commonly in young children between the ages of 2 and 6 years with a secondary peak, of predominantly paratesticular rhabdomyosarcoma, in teenagers. Genitourinary and retroperitoneal tumors account for between 20 and 30% of all rhabdomyosarcomas [3].

Genitourinary rhabdomyosarcomas include those tumors arising in the bladder, prostate, spermatic cord, epididymis, testes, penis, vagina and uterus. In the female, the two most common locations are the base of the bladder and high in the wall of the vagina. In the male, the tumors occur commonly in the bladder, prostate or scrotum. The term paratesticular rhabdomyosarcoma is used to designate those tumors arising in the scrotum [2]. This term is needed because it is frequently impossible to determine whether the tumor has actually arisen from the testes, the tunica, the epididymis, or the spermatic cord. Clinical symptoms of genitourinary rhabdomyosarcoma are nonspecific and include urinary retention, dysuria, hematuria, fecal retention, or a palpable or visible mass. Metastases occur in order of decreasing frequency to lymph nodes, lung, liver, bone, bone marrow, soft tissue and central nervous system.

Paratesticular rhabdomyosarcomas are usually treated with initial surgical resection followed by chemotherapy and have an overall survival of about 80%. Bladder, prostatic, and vaginal rhabdomyosarcomas are now being treated with initial aggressive chemotherapy followed by delayed attempted complete surgical resection of residual tumor without causing unacceptable damage to vital organs and structures. Radiation therapy may be given as well. Overall survival for these tumors is about 60%.

Table 1. Common pelvic tumors in children

Tumor type	Percentage of all tumors of this type occurring in the pelvis or gonads
Germ cell	90
Rhabdomyosarcoma	15-30
Ewing sarcoma	10-20
Neuroblastoma	5

Table 2. Classification of testicular tumors in children

- Primary malignant tumors of the testis
  Germ cell tumors (70%)
  Stromal tumors (20%)
  Gonadoblastoma (5%)
  Other (5%)
- Paratesticular tumors
  Rhabdomyosarcoma
- Metastatic tumors
  Leukemia
  Lymphoma
  Neuroblastoma
  Wilms' tumor

Ewing Sarcoma of the Pelvis

Ewing sarcoma is the second most common malignant bone tumor in children [2]. The pelvis is the second most common site for this tumor with between 10% and 20% of Ewing sarcomas occurring in the pelvis. The pathology and behavior of this tumor is not site-specific with pelvic tumors having similar histology and patterns of metastases to those in other locations. Common sites for metastases include lung, other bones, and lymph nodes. Pain is the commonest presenting symptom. The tumors most typically arise in the iliac bone, demonstrate extensive bone destruction and frequently have a large soft tissue mass at the time of presentation. Bone marrow spread as identified on magnetic resonance imaging is frequently more extensive than one would anticipate from evaluation of the bone cortex destruction. Pelvic Ewing sarcomas have a poorer prognosis than Ewing's sarcomas occurring at other sites.

Germ Cell Tumors

These are the commonest primary tumors of the testes. Before discussing the germ cell tumors of the testes it is worth reviewing the pathophysiology of these tumors in general [2].

Germ cell tumors are uncommon and their histologic classification is complicated, with considerable disagreement existing [4]. In addition to there being a wide range of different histologic tumors, they may occur at many different sites in the body, and the behavior and appearance of the tumors will vary considerably depending on the anatomic location. There is also confusion with regard to the definition of malignancy. Some initially benign tumors may recur as a malignant tumor. Other tumors may contain both benign and malignant elements. Germ cell tumors account for approximately 3% of all pediatric cancers. The most common age of presentation and the sex difference with these tumors are summarized in Table 3.

The pathology of germ cell tumors is interesting. Germ cell tumor is an all-embracing term and includes a variety of different tumors linked together because of overlapping histology and common origin [4]. All germ cell tumors arise from primordial germ cells of the yolk sac that normally migrate to the gonads but can have their migration arrested along the route of passage or may occasionally occur in ectopic sites. Most of these tumors are always malignant but some, for example a teratoma, may be benign (mature) or malignant. Most malignant teratomas contain tissues of other types of germ cell tumor. Some publications will call these lesions malignant teratomas, while most authorities would classify them by the more malignant tissue. For example, a teratoma showing areas of endodermal sinus tumor would be called an endodermal sinus tumor. One of the more

widely accepted classifications of germ cell tumors is presented in Table 4. The following points should be noted [5]:

- Only teratomas and yolk sac tumors occur in children with any significant frequency.
- The term yolk sac tumor is synonymous with endodermal sinus tumor. Most would include infantile embryonal carcinoma with yolk sac tumor.
- Germinoma has previously been called seminoma in the testicle and dysgerminoma in the ovary. The term germinoma should be used for these tumors regardless of site.
- Adult embryonal carcinoma almost never occurs in children.
- Most testicular tumors are pure yolk sac.

Table 3. Germ cell tumors: age and sex epidemiology

Tumor type	Sex differences	Age
Sacrococcygeal teratoma	80% female	Mostly newborn
Yolk sac: testis	All male	80% under 2 years
Retroperitoneal teratoma	75% female	50% under 6 months Mean 5 months
Ovarian teratoma	All female	Puberty

Table 4. Histologic classification of germ cell tumors [4]

Teratoma
  Mature
  Immature
Germinoma
Adult embryonal carcinoma
Yolk sac tumor (endodermal sinus tumor)
Choriocarcinoma
Gonadoblastoma
Mixed germ cell

Table 5. Likelihood of malignancy in pediatric germ cell tumors

Anatomic site	Likelihood of malignancy

Sacrococcygeal	Age dependent
	  Newborn-1 month 2% malignant
	  Over 1 month 71% malignant
	  Overall 13% malignant

Testis	Over 80% malignant
Ovary	Over 60% benign
Head and neck	Usually benign
Vagina	Usually malignant
Retroperitoneum	< 10% malignant
Gastric	All benign
Anterior mediastinum	20% malignant

Table 6. Classification of sacrococcygeal teratoma and likelihood of malignancy

Stage		Incidence (%)	Malignancy (%)
I	Predominantly external	49	8
II	External with pelvic component	34	21
III	External with pelvic and abdominal component	8.0	34
IV	Presacral (no external component)	9.0	38

Table 7. Survival of 126 children with malignant germ cell tumors [5]

By site			By stage		
	No.	Survival (%)		No.	Survival (%)
Testis	59	100	I	62	97
Vagina, uterus, prostate	4	100	II	14	86
			III	18	83
Ovary	25	88	IV	16	72
Thorax	5	40			

Not all germ cell tumors are malignant. Most teratomas are benign. All yolk sac tumors should be considered malignant. The likelihood of a germ cell tumor being malignant is very much dependent on its anatomic site (Tables 5, 6).

Staging of germ cell tumors is a problem and it is important for the radiologist to be aware that there is no universally accepted staging system. Some institutions adopt different staging systems for different anatomic locations of the tumor. One classification that has been used for some collaborative studies is presented in Table 6.

Clinically, most germ cell tumors present with signs and symptoms of the local tumor mass [2, 6]. Presentation with diffuse metastatic disease is decidedly uncommon. The presenting symptoms are varied, reflecting the multitude of anatomic locations of the primary tumor. Sacrococcygeal teratomas most often present as an easily detectable exophytic mass that is almost always very large [7]. In the small number of sacrococcygeal teratomas in which the tumor is entirely presacral, the diagnosis may be delayed and symptoms will include difficulty with urination or defecation or urinary infection. Testicular tumors most often present as a painless mass. Attention is occasionally drawn to the mass by accidental trauma.

Tumor markers are important in the management of germ cell tumors. Alpha-fetoprotein is an alpha 1 globulin and is the main normally occurring serum protein in the fetus. It has a halflife of about 5 days. Its concentration in the serum is increased in patients with hepatomas, hepatitis, some gastrointestinal tumors, and yolk sac tumors. It is not increased with dysgerminomas, choriocarcinomas, or mature teratomas. It is reliably and consistently elevated in patients with yolk sac tumors. The degree of elevation of alpha-fetoprotein has no relationship to tumor prognosis. The finding of elevated alpha-fetoprotein is very helpful; however, in the differential diagnosis of a tumor. It is also extremely helpful to serially measure concentrations of alpha-fetoprotein after therapy. Levels return to normal with satisfactory response to therapy and become elevated very quickly with tumor relapse.

Therapy and prognosis. Prior to the 1960s malignant germ cell tumors, with the exception of those that could initially be completely resected, were uniformly fatal. With the introduction of chemotherapy, prognosis has improved considerably. In the pre-1980 era, it improved to approximately 42% overall. For many of these tumors the prognosis is extremely good (Table 7). The prognosis is best for the genitourinary primary tumors and not as good in other locations [5]. The prognosis is not dependent on the tumor histology and is the same for pure yolk sac tumors as it is for yolk sac tumor mixed with teratoma.

With regard to therapy, radiation therapy is little utilized in the frontline management of germ cell tumors. Surgical excision of all tumors is performed when possible. Most patients are treated with both surgery and chemotherapy. The only exception to this is stage I testicular yolk sac tumor for which surgery alone can be curative.

Gonadoblastoma [2]

These tumors are mixed germ cell and stromal tumors. They occur only in dysgenetic gonads in children with associated chromosome abnormalities and true or pseudo hermaphroditism. One-third are bilateral and they may produce estrogen. The stromal component of these tumors is almost always benign. The germ cell component may be malignant.

Stromal Tumors of the Testes [8]

Leydig cell tumors are the most common gonadal stromal tumors. They produce androgens and cause precocious puberty. The peak age of presentation is at about 4 years. They are invariably benign and do not metastasize, and treatment is by local surgical excision [9].

Sertoli cell tumors have a peak incidence at 18 months. They usually present as a testicular mass with or without signs of precocious puberty. The masses are usually small at the time of diagnosis and treatment is by surgical excision. These tumors are usually benign.

Lymphoma and Leukemia of the Testes

Leukemic involvement usually does not occur at initial presentation, but after initial induction therapy. Microscopically both testes are usually involved, although clinically it is common for only one testicle to be enlarged. Imaging findings are nonspecific and biopsy is usually needed for confirmation of diagnosis. The testes may rarely be the site for lymphoma, usually Burkitt's lymphoma.

Suggested Reading

1. Barth RA, Teele RL, Colodny A, et al. (1984) Asymptomatic scrotal masses in children. Radiology 152: 65-68
2. Cohen MD (1992) Imaging of children with cancer. Mosby Year Book, St. Louis
3. La Quaglia MP (1996) Genitourinary tract cancer in childhood. Sem Pediatr Surg 1: 49-65
4. Dehner LP (1983) Gonadal and extragonadal germ cell neoplasia of childhood. Hum Pathol 14: 493-511
5. Mann JR, Pearson D, Barrett A, et al. (1989) Results of the United Kingdom Children's Cancer Study Group's Malignant Germ Cell Tumor Studies. Cancer 63: 1657-1667
6. Kaplan GW, Cromie WC, Kelalis PP, et al. (1988) Prepubertal yolk sac testicular tumors-report of the testicular tumor registry. J Urol 140: 1109-1112
7. Noseworthy J, Lack EE, Kozakewich HPW, et al. (1981) Sacrococcygeal germ cell tumors in childhood: an updated experience with 118 patients. J Pediatr Surg 16: 358-364
8. Fernandes ET, Etcubanas E, Bar BN, et al. (1989) Two decades of experience with testicular tumors in children at St Jude Children's Research Hospital. J Pediatr Surg 24: 677-682
9. Exelby PR (1980) Testicular cancer in children. Cancer 45: 1803-1809

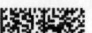